Homeopathy at Home

Homeopathy at Home

Everyday Treatments for Common Complaints

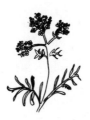

MARCUS FERNANDEZ

Founder, Centre for Homeopathic Education

HAY HOUSE

Carlsbad, California • New York City
London • Sydney • New Delhi

Published in the United Kingdom by:
Hay House UK Ltd, 1st Floor, Crawford Corner
91–93 Baker Street, London W1U 6QQ
Tel: +44 (0)20 3927 7290; www.hayhouse.co.uk

Published in the United States of America by:
Hay House LLC, PO Box 5100, Carlsbad, CA 92018-5100
Tel: (1) 760 431 7695 or (800) 654 5126; www.hayhouse.com

Published in Australia by:
Hay House Australia Publishing Pty Ltd, 18/36 Ralph St, Alexandria NSW 2015
Tel: (61) 2 9669 4299; www.hayhouse.com.au

Published in India by:
Hay House Publishers (India) Pvt Ltd, Muskaan Complex,
Plot No.3, B-2, Vasant Kunj, New Delhi 110 070
Tel: (91) 11 4176 1620; www.hayhouse.co.in

A catalogue record for this book is available from the British Library.

Tradepaper ISBN: 978-1-4019-8024-5
E-book ISBN: 978-1-83782-320-8

Interior images: Shutterstock

10 9 8 7 6 5 4 3 2 1

Printed in the United States of America

This product uses responsibly sourced papers and/or recycled materials. For more information, see www.hayhouse.com.

This book is dedicated to Dr Robin Murphy ND,
my teacher, my inspiration and my friend.

*'The natural healing force within each of us
is the greatest force in getting well.'*
HIPPOCRATES

CONTENTS

Contents

INTRODUCTION

I didn't find homeopathy; it found me.

I was not brought up with homeopathy; if I was sick, my mum would take me to the doctor, and I'd take whatever drug was prescribed. I was taken to chickenpox parties and had all the typical childhood diseases and vaccinations. However, even from an early age, I didn't like taking medicines; it didn't feel right and I often felt worse afterwards.

At 20 years old, I was living my dream as the lead singer of a rock/punk band. We had a single out and were just about to go on a small tour in Germany. Being a struggling musician, I needed to earn some money to bring with me, as we only got paid once we'd done a gig. The only job I could get was working in a nursing home for the elderly. Working in the care industry was the last thing on my mind but I told myself it would only be temporary, and then I'd be back on my way to making it big in the music industry!

I'd only been working at the care home for a couple of weeks when one of the nurses struck up a conversation with me during my coffee break. We chatted for a while, and then, out of the blue, she said to me, *'You know what? You'd make a good homeopath.'* I had absolutely no idea what she was talking about; I didn't even know what the word meant! She explained what it was and told me she was starting a four-year training course to become a homeopath. She was going to an open day for the course and asked me to join her. I was a bit flummoxed by her invitation, since I'd already told her about my rock-'n'-roll aspirations! I politely declined and left the break room but, in the days that followed, she kept trying to persuade me to go along. Eventually, I agreed to go with her but made it quite clear that it was only to shut her up! I had no intention of signing up for the course!

As a singer, I suffered from recurrent tonsillitis. I was living an unhealthy lifestyle, having late nights and spending my time in smoky pubs. Whenever I got sick, I'd make a trip to the doctor to get a course of antibiotics without a second thought. On the day before the open day, I woke up with terrible tonsillitis. I couldn't get an appointment with the doctor, so I thought I'd try a homeopathic remedy instead. I caught the bus into town and went to the local natural health store. I found a selection of homeopathic remedies at the back of the store, and started looking for a remedy that might help with my tonsillitis.

There were very strange names on the bottles, like 'Calc Carb' and 'Hepar Sulph' – they sounded like something from a chemistry class. I thought 'Nux Vomica' would make a great name for a heavy rock band! I picked up a leaflet that explained what condition each remedy could help with. The remedy 'Gelsemium' fitted my symptoms: 'shooting pains in ears, made worse by swallowing; apathetic; heavy, droopy eyelids; a headache that feels like a tight band around the head'. That sounded like me.

I bought the remedy and decided that if it worked, I would go to the open day, and if it didn't, I wouldn't. I felt sleepy not long after taking the remedy, so I took a short nap... for three hours! When I woke up, I was soaked in sweat. *Wow*, I thought, *this stuff is powerful.*

I took the remedy throughout the rest of the day and continued to sweat profusely. I woke up the next morning with no tonsillitis! It was remarkable.

I was so impressed. This remedy had a deep healing effect on my body and not only had my tonsillitis gone, but I felt clearer and more energetic than I had for a long time. I kept the promise to myself and went with my new friend to the open day at the homeopathic college. (By the way, I haven't had another bout of tonsillitis in 32 years!)

When the late, great Robert Davidson spoke at the open day and shared his knowledge and clinical experience of homeopathy, I experienced a stillness within me that I'd never felt before. It felt like I was hearing 'truth' for the very first time. I was transfixed; it resonated deeply within my being. My first thought was, *If this is true, why doesn't the whole world know about it?* And without hesitation, my second thought was, *I'm going to make sure the whole world* does *know about it!*

Homeopathy had found me.

That day marked the beginning of an amazing journey spanning 33 years. Homeopathy has taken me all over the world, teaching and practising, from the skyscrapers of New York to under a tree in a remote African village. Through my homeopathic school, The Centre for Homeopathic Education, we've trained some fantastic students who have become great practitioners, spreading the light of homoeopathy around the globe.

There are very few things in life that can have a real impact on people's lives – homeopathy is one of them.

My aim is to enhance the health and wellbeing of humankind through the use of homeopathy. I wanted to write a simple and accessible guide to managing common acute and minor complaints using homeopathic remedies at home. I want people to feel empowered. We all have innate health. Homoeopathic remedies act like keys to a lock – choose the correct key and it turns the lock, stimulating the body to heal itself. It's good to remember that the body has a natural healing wisdom; we just need to turn the key and remind it what it needs to do.

This book is organized as an A–Z list of common complaints and briefly explains each condition and the best remedies. There's also a section on other home remedies, commonly found in most kitchens, that can be used alongside the recommended homeopathic remedy.

There's no better way to learn homeopathy than by practising it: taking (or giving) the remedy and seeing the effects. Start practising with simple first-aid problems such as minor cuts, burns and bruises until you're familiar with how the remedies work. Nearly everyone experiences the same symptoms with first-aid injuries, so it's easy to learn which remedy to give for each situation. For example, in the case of bruising following an impact, Arnica is a go-to remedy.

As your confidence grows, start practising on acute complaints such as coughs, colds and headaches, where it's much more important to focus on an individual's symptoms. For example, with a cold, symptoms can vary from person to person. Therefore, the remedies used should be chosen for the individual.

What is health?

Many people's concept of health is *not being sick*, but it's so much more than that. Health is about *vitality*, the sense of feeling alive mentally, emotionally and physically. I remember when I was a child, I'd be out all day on my bike during the school holidays. I'd come home, eat, sleep and leap out of bed the next morning, ready to do it all over again with enthusiasm, a sense of adventure and a zest for life. This is vitality. Most children have a strong vitality and embrace life with enthusiasm, wonder and being in the moment. Often, if they're sick with an acute illness, they may have a fever or vomit, but the next day, they're up eating their breakfast, ready for the next adventure!

What is dis-ease?

Health is about our ability to adapt to our environment. This could be a physical or emotional adaptation, such as a change between seasons or losing a loved one. Our resilience against illness depends on our vitality and susceptibility. These determine whether we become sick or unwell and our ability to recover.

Symptoms are the body's way of saying, 'Hey, there's a problem here.' If we don't listen to the body at this point, we'll be forced to listen when it falters. If we suppress the symptoms, we're simply pushing the issue further into the body, which might result in a more chronic condition later.

Let's use a car dashboard as an example. The oil light flashes, which means there's something wrong with the engine; if we take the bulb out to stop the light flashing, there's still a problem with the engine, and the car may break down a few miles down the road. In homeopathy, we see the symptom as the oil light flashing, so we go into the engine and fix the cause. Then, the oil light will no longer flash: the 'symptom' disappears.

Our susceptibility is constantly changing. Think of it as a scale. When you wake up in the morning after a good night's sleep, your vitality might be at 8/10. Then, you open the post and get a shock; you have a large utility bill you weren't expecting, and your vitality goes down to 6/10. You're running late, miss the bus and must walk to the office in heavy rain. By the time you get to work, your vitality is down to 4/10. A colleague has a cold, so it's no surprise that by the end of the day, you're feeling unwell, too. Your lowered vitality made you more susceptible to catching a bug. Not everyone at your work goes home coughing and sneezing, just those with low vitality and increased susceptibility.

The homeopathic approach

Most conventional medications focus on relieving symptoms rather than addressing the underlying cause. In contrast, in homeopathy we see the symptoms as the body's attempt to heal itself – perhaps needing help but of a gentle and supportive kind. Homeopathy treats an individual with a specific set of symptoms, focusing on *why* a remedy is being given rather than *what* remedy is given.

Homeopathy is a whole system of medicine that looks at each person holistically – physically, mentally and emotionally. It's not about treating the symptoms, but about understanding the individual and their unique experience of the disease. It's not just about what you have, but about how and why you have it.

For example, five people could receive a diagnosis of 'Influenza', but each person may experience different symptoms. One person might be thirsty for ice-cold water, while another would prefer warm drinks. One person may feel hot, while another feels chilly. One might have headaches, and another may experience pain in their bones.

In homeopathy, we don't use a one-size-fits-all approach. Before recommending a remedy, we consider the totality of an individual's experience of disease by gathering information and asking questions: what makes the symptoms worse or better, when the symptoms started, what was happening at the time, where the pain or symptom is located and so on.

Homeopathy comes from the Greek words 'homeo', meaning similar, and 'pathos', meaning suffering. The German doctor Samuel Hahnemann founded the principle of homeopathy around the end of the 18th century and developed it as a system of medicine that we still use and follow today.

Hahnemann was disillusioned with the medical practices of the day, with crude drug therapy doing more harm than good to patients. He left medical practice and became a translator. While translating a medical book from English to German, he came across a claim about Cinchona Bark being used for treating Malaria. As a scientist, he was sceptical of the claim and decided to test the bark on himself to observe its effects. What he discovered was that he began to develop the symptoms of Malaria. When he stopped the treatment, the symptoms disappeared. He carried on experimenting with other substances and concluded that a remedy's therapeutic potential lies in its ability to produce effects on the body. Paradoxically, the same substance that can cause symptoms in a healthy person may alleviate similar symptoms in someone who is ill.

There are three main principles of homeopathy:

- Like cures like
- One remedy at a time
- The minimum dose

Like cures like

The concept of *like cures like,* or the Law of Similars, is not new; it goes back 2,500 years. Hippocrates is thought to have said, 'By similar things a disease is produced and through the application of the like is cured,' meaning a substance capable of causing the symptoms of a disease can also cure it; a remedy acts as a stimulus for the body's natural healing response, providing the support it needs to carry out the healing process.

A good example of *like cures like* involves the common onion. Chopping an onion can often cause the eyes to water and the nose to run. These same symptoms can be experienced by individuals who have a cold or hay fever. Allium Cepa, made from red onion, is used in homoeopathy to treat these symptoms. Another example is coffee. Drinking too much coffee can cause restlessness, jitters and sleep disturbance. In homeopathy, Coffea Cruda, prepared from coffee, is a remedy used to help people experiencing insomnia or nervous excitement.

So, a substance that can cause symptoms in a healthy person can, in small, diluted doses, treat similar symptoms in someone feeling unwell by stimulating the body's healing force.

One remedy at a time

When considering a remedy for acute conditions, the aim is to match the remedy's characteristics to the totality of the symptoms presented. 'Totality' is a homeopathic term meaning the whole picture, including a person's mental, emotional and physical symptoms. For example, Bryonia may be a remedy for someone with a hot, sore, swollen ankle who is thirsty for cold water, is irritable and wants to be left alone.

To see clearly how a remedy is working, it's better to give one remedy at a time. Give a single dose, wait and assess the effects of the remedy, and repeat if the symptoms return. It may be necessary to repeat the dose frequently in first-aid situations. Sometimes a combination remedy, where several remedies are taken together, is appropriate – for example, teething or hay fever. The drawback is that the combination may work for a while, but if it stops working, it may be unclear which remedy within the combination helped, making it difficult to increase the dose of that remedy if needed.

The minimum dose

In homeopathy, remedies are diluted to very small amounts to stimulate the body's innate healing potential. The aim is to use the least stimulus possible to restore health and wellbeing, not high, concentrated doses that come with possible side effects. Once the remedy gently stimulates the body's own healing capability, it doesn't need to be repeated unless the symptoms start to return or stop improving.

FINDING AND PRESCRIBING THE CORRECT REMEDY

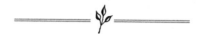

Identifying each person's individual symptoms is key to guiding the choice of remedy specific to that person's symptoms. For example, one person has a headache that feels like a tight band around the head. The headache is a dull, heavy ache that appeared after receiving bad news. Here, the remedy would be Gelsemium. Another person has a headache with pain at the back of the head that spreads over their eyes. They're suffering from a hangover after a night out when they consumed a lot of alcohol. They can be very irritable, want to be alone and feel nauseous. The remedy in this case would be Nux Vomica.

Type of complaint

When considering homeopathy, it's important to determine if the condition is acute or chronic.

- **Acute** illnesses are self-limiting and characterized by rapid onset, a clear pattern, a definite end and an expectation of complete recovery. For example, influenza.

- **Chronic** illnesses typically come with symptoms that don't clear up, may change in nature and get worse over time. For example, irritable bowel syndrome (IBS).

Homeopathy at Home provides remedies for acute conditions, not chronic illnesses. For chronic conditions, please seek the services of a qualified professional homeopath (*see Resources on page 245*).

Getting the information: CLAMS

A quick way to get the most relevant information in order to select the appropriate remedy is to use the CLAMS method:

- **C**oncomitant (symptoms that accompany the main complaint)
- **L**ocation (where the pain/symptom is located within the body)
- **A**etiology (the possible cause behind the complaint)
- **M**odalities (what makes the complaint better or worse)
- **S**ensation (what is the pain like, e.g. sore, shooting)

Write the abbreviations 'CLAMS' vertically down one side of a sheet of paper. Then, fill in the information about the symptoms of the complaint. Once you have this information, you can identify the closest-matching remedy.

Example

A person has a dry, hacking cough that's so painful and sore they must hold their chest each time they cough. This symptom started after being outdoors and exposed to cold wind. The cough is worse when they come into a warm room and better when they are still. The person is very thirsty, irritable and wants to be alone.

- **C**: irritable, thirsty, wants to be left alone

- **L**: lungs

- **A**: cold wind

- **M**: worse with movement and in a warm room; better when still

- **S**: dry, soreness and pain

Turn to the 'Coughs' entry to find nine possible remedies (*see page 67*). In this case, Bryonia is the closest-matching cough remedy to the symptoms described above. The symptoms described are highlighted in bold.

Bryonia

- Slow, **gradual onset**; hard, **dry, hacking, painful** cough; **irritability of upper trachea** (windpipe); **holds chest to keep it still**; **soreness** with sharp, **stabbing pains** in sides of chest; **dry throat** with very little phlegm; **irritable**; very **thirsty**, drinks in large gulps; headaches

- Cough causes the individual to involuntarily leap from their bed or chair

- Worse from **movement**; talking; laughing; **entering a warm room**; inhaling; at night

- Better from **being still**; cool, **open air**; resting; lying on painful side; with **hard pressure**; having cold drinks

Using the CLAMS method helps you to identify the most important symptoms so you can select the right remedy.

Understanding keynotes

Once you have gathered the main information using the CLAMS method, you can then match the detailed symptoms to the correct remedy. Each homeopathic remedy has a vast clinical picture with many symptoms, so it's helpful to understand the concept of keynotes. The **keynotes** in homeopathy are the distinctive characteristics of a remedy that enable you to identify it quickly and accurately. They act as signposts to a remedy and have, over time, proven to be the most reliable characteristics of that remedy. Think of keynotes as the unique signature or fingerprint of a remedy.

One remedy can have several keynotes. Some remedies have more keynotes than others. To select a remedy, it's helpful to look for a minimum of three keynotes – symptoms that stand out right away. I like to think of this like a well-known song – you hear the first three notes and immediately know what the song is. It's the same with homeopathy: the three characteristic symptoms (keynotes) tell you what remedy is needed. This technique is commonly referred to in homeopathy as using the 'three-legged stool'. The keynotes can help identify a particular remedy quickly; they act like flags for a remedy.

For instance, let's imagine you go to the gym and wake up the next day feeling stiff. The stiffness is **worse** with the **first movement** but **gets better** with **continued movement** and **heat**, such as a hot bath. Although there may be other characteristics, these three are the keynotes – the 'legs' of the stool – and make it easier to identify Rhus Tox as the appropriate remedy.

Each remedy has unique keynotes that differentiate it from others, even those with similar therapeutic effects. For example, Rhus Tox and Bryonia are both used for joint pain, but Rhus Tox is recommended when the pain **gets better** with **continued movement**, while Bryonia is recommended when the pain gets **worse** with **any movement**. This distinction is important when choosing the appropriate remedy.

Keynotes are not limited physical symptoms. They can also include mental and emotional states. For instance, the remedy Ignatia is often given for grief and emotional distress. Its keynotes include a sensation of a lump in the throat and much sighing. These emotional keynotes are just as important as the physical ones in creating a complete picture of the remedy.

The advantage of using keynotes is that they simplify the process of home prescribing by focusing on standout symptoms. This allows for more accurate and effective choices for acute conditions.

Let's use hay fever as another example of how using keynotes can be helpful. While three people exhibit hay fever symptoms, each person may require a different remedy:

- Person A experiences a runny nose, but the main symptom is red eyes with watery tears that cause a burning sensation, which is made worse by being in a warm room.

- Person B has symptoms that also affect the eyes; however, they feel like they have sand in their eyes and have a headache across their forehead.

- Person C experiences a lot of sneezing and pronounced itching in the nose, throat and roof of the mouth.

These three people experience their hay fever symptoms differently. Matching their standout symptoms and to a remedy's keynotes can help find the most effective homeopathic medicine.

The **emboldened text** under each remedy in this guidebook indicates the keynotes.

Choosing a remedy and dose

Select the remedy that best matches the most distinct symptoms, rather than the most common ones. For example, if someone has a cold with a runny nose, the runny nose is a common symptom. However, if the discharge causes a burning sensation to the nose and upper lip, and their eyes are light-sensitive, these are more distinct symptoms and would suggest the remedy Allium Cepa. To find the best remedy, identify the keynotes: at least three characteristic symptoms.

After writing down the symptoms using the CLAMS method (*see page xxii*), compare them with the remedies under that complaint in this book. Give a single dose of the chosen remedy, either in tablet or capsule form. Homeopathic medicines can be bought online or over the counter at health stores and pharmacies. They are usually in a 6c or 30c potency, a good choice for most acute conditions. Higher potencies should be left to qualified homeopathic prescribers.

Cell salts, also known as tissue salts, are sometimes mentioned in this book, too, for different health issues. These usually come in a 6x potency. Rather than treating 'like with like', these remedies manage conditions by helping the body restore itself through correcting imbalances or deficiencies.

For some people and situations, such as treating babies or young children, remedies can come in different forms, and these can also be ordered via a homoeopathic pharmacy. Ask for advice if you're not sure which remedy or form is best suited to you.

Give one dose, wait for a couple of hours and observe how you or the person being treated feels. Often, children will fall asleep after a dose, which can be a good sign that the body has started the healing process. If you or the person being treated feels much better after a dose, stop taking the remedy until the symptoms return. Then, the remedy can be repeated.

Repeating the remedy

There's no set protocol for when to repeat the remedy. The best approach is to be guided by how you or the person being treated feels and the severity of the symptoms. For instance, in first-aid scenarios like a nosebleed, it may be necessary to repeat the remedy every five minutes until the bleeding stops. Similarly, for a high fever, the remedy may need to be taken every half-hour. Remember, less is more; the remedy acts as a stimulus to get the body to start the healing process. The body knows what to do.

As I mentioned before, a remedy acts like a key. Think about a key to a car. The key is used to turn on the ignition to start the engine. This action doesn't need to be repeated unless the engine stops. It's the same with a homeopathic remedy – once it gently stimulates the body's own healing capability, it doesn't need to be repeated unless the symptoms start to return or stop improving.

The individualized homeopathic approach is significantly different from the standard pharmaceutical protocol, which typically requires people to complete a full course of medication or to follow a strict dosing schedule.

Can homeopathic remedies be taken with prescription drugs?

There are no known reports of cross-reactions with conventional medical treatments. If you're unsure, speak to the prescribing doctor or contact a homeopathic pharmacy.

Are homeopathic remedies safe?

Homeopathic remedies are safe and free from side effects because they work differently to conventional medication. They're safe for use during pregnancy and for babies and young children, who often respond more quickly to homeopathic treatments than adults.

How should I take the remedies?

Most homeopathic medicines come in small tablets that should be dissolved or chewed in a clean mouth. If possible, do not handle the tablets directly; instead, tip them into the bottle cap and then into your mouth.

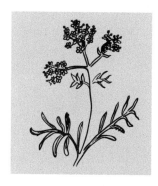
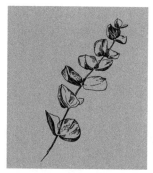
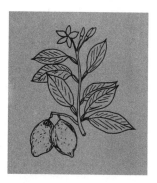

A–Z OF COMMON
COMPLAINTS

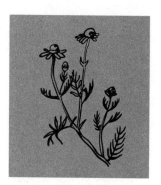
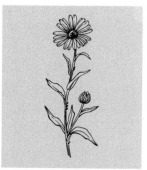
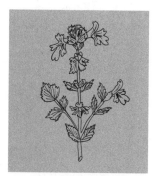

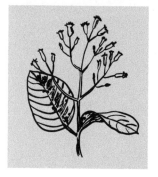
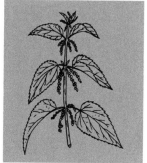
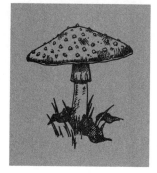

ACNE

Acne is an indication of hormonal surges or fluctuations within the body. It is most experienced by teenagers but can occur later in life, too, especially in women during times of hormonal change, such as menstruation, ovulation, pregnancy or menopause. Due to overactivity of the sebaceous glands, hair follicles become blocked with oil and dead skin cells.

Signs of acne include:

- Skin eruptions on the face, back, chest or shoulders

- Blackheads (dark spots on the skin)

- Whiteheads (closed white or yellow bumps on the skin)

- Pimples (small red bumps that are sensitive and sore)

- Pustules (like pimples but with a pus-filled centre)

- Nodules (large, hard, painful lumps under the surface of the skin)

- Cysts (pus-filled lumps that can lead to scarring)

Actions that may help:

- Avoid washing the skin more than twice a day to prevent irritation.
- Use non-oil-based makeup and skincare products.
- Eat a balanced, wholefood diet and stay hydrated.
- Maintain a good sleep routine, with focus on quality and length of sleep.
- Practise mindfulness or meditation to reduce stress.

HOMEOPATHIC REMEDIES

Kali Brom

- **Purplish** acne; **scarring**; large, **painful**, **burning**, **stinging** or **itching** pustules
- Acne of the face (cheeks and forehead), chest and **shoulders**
- Worse around **puberty**; **menstruation**
- Better in **cold** weather

Silica

- **Deep**, **hard** cystic pimples; **eruptions that are slow to heal**; skin prone to **scarring**; the individual often feels **cold**; **sweaty** hands and feet
- Pimples may appear in **crops** and turn into boils with **pus**
- Worse when exposed to **cold air**; when **sweat is suppressed**
- Better during the **summer**; when **warm**

Silica helps in expelling foreign bodies and pus from the skin and promotes the healing of acne scars.

Sulphur

- **Red**, **inflamed** pimples and blackheads; **oily** skin
- Skin may **itch** and **burn** when scratched
- Worse with **heat**; **washing**
- Better after **sweating**; in **open air**

Calc Sulph 6x

This cell salt is good for acne on the face, including pimples and pustules with a yellow discharge and crusts. The skin heals slowly and is very sensitive to touch.

Kali Sulph 6x

This cell salt is useful in managing acne that presents with either thin, dark yellow, weeping discharge or thick and sticky discharge. Also acne that is worse around menstruation.

OTHER HOME REMEDIES

Tea tree oil

Tea tree oil is a good choice to help reduce and heal acne. It has antibacterial and anti-inflammatory properties. Don't put the oil directly onto the skin; instead mix a few drops with a carrier oil (such as almond, olive or coconut) so the tea tree oil is less likely to irritate the skin.

Honey and cinnamon mask

Mix two tablespoons of honey with one teaspoon of Ceylon cinnamon powder to make a paste. Apply to the face to reduce inflammation and kill unwanted bacteria.

Green tea

Green tea helps regulate the sebaceous glands. Using a cotton wool pad, apply cooled green tea to the face or use the tea as a face wash.

ANXIETY

Anxiety is characterized by an uneasy feeling of fear, dread or apprehension of what is likely to happen; overreactions to possible or imagined events in the future with an uncertain outcome; or excessive and unrealistic worry about the consequences of future events.

Signs of anxiety include:

- Feeling very tense

- Nervousness

- Being restless and agitated

- A sense of impending danger or immediate threat

Anxiety may result in a panic attack with physical symptoms including:

- Increased heart rate

- Excessive sweating

- Rapid breathing

- Trembling

- An inability to think about anything else

Actions that may help:

- Practise mindfulness or meditation, either at home or by joining a class.

- Try breath regulation using a deep-breathing technique. Inhale slowly through your nose for four counts and exhale slowly through your mouth for four counts. Do this for five minutes.

- Regular exercise can help reduce anxiety by releasing endorphins and promoting a sense of wellbeing.

- Try journalling to express your thoughts and feelings. Writing can help you process emotions, gain clarity and reduce anxiety.

Experimenting with different strategies and finding what works best for you is important. If anxiety persists or significantly interferes with daily functioning, consider seeking professional help.

HOMEOPATHIC REMEDIES

Aconite

- Intense, **sudden onset** of anxiety, **panic** or **fear**; dry skin; **dry mouth**; **tingling** of the mouth, tongue and limbs; **fast heartbeat**; sense of **foreboding** and fear of **imminent death**

- Can be connected to **past trauma**, **fright** or **shock**

- Worse at night, especially around **midnight**

- Better from exposure to **open air**; with **rest**

Argent Nit

- Fear of **losing control**; hypochondria; **catastrophizing**; **claustrophobia**; fear of heights or flying; **impulsive**; impatient; **sweet cravings**; **digestive disturbance**, e.g. diarrhoea

- Can be due to feelings of uncertainty or **anticipation** before an event, e.g. going to an appointment, giving a talk, taking an exam

- Worse in closed, **small places**; in crowds; from **warmth**; when **apprehensive**; from eating sugar

- Better with exposure to cool, **open air**; from taking **cold baths**; with **movement**

Arsenicum Album

- **Restlessness** with anxiety about health, finances or exposure to dirt and germs; very fearful and difficult to reassure; **hopeless** about recovery; dreads death; **fastidious**; very **chilly**; **thirsty** for sips of cold water; desperate for company; **controlling** or **critical** of others

- Worse with **physical exertion**; between **11 p.m. and 2 a.m.**; from exposure to **cold air**; from eating **cold food**

- Better with **heat**; company; **warm drinks**

Gelsemium

- Feelings of **anticipation**; **speechless**; nervous; **shaky**; **agoraphobic** or fear of crowds; **weakness**; trembling; feeling faint; gas or diarrhoea; apathetic; desires **solitude**

- Can be due to anticipation of an event, such as public speaking or being in the spotlight, or fear of failure, e.g. exams

- Worse following **bad news**; from anticipation; when **frightened**; from thinking about the condition

- Better in the **afternoon**; with **continued motion**; after **urinating**

Ignatia

- Feeling that something terrible has happened; sensation of **lump in throat**; **sighing**; generally **feeling down**; **oversensitive**; prone to **mood swings**; fear of house burglary at night; fear of being **hurt** and **disappointed**

- Can be due to **grief**, **disappointment** or **loss**; an emotional shock; a **fright** with hysteria and **crying**

- Worse with **coffee** or stimulants

- Better for **being alone**

Lycopodium

- Lacks **self-confidence**; fear of **failure** or being **inadequate**; **panic attacks**; churning stomach; **angry**; **irritable**; digestive issues, e.g. **gas** and **bloating**

- Anxiety about **responsibilities** or **performance**; will take it out on others

- Better for **walking** in **open air**

- Worse from **being alone**

Phosphorus

- Excessive **worrying**; **oversensitive** to atmospheres, people, news; **overactive mind** and imagination; **scattered thoughts**; **restlessness**; panic attacks; **hyperventilation**; fear of thunderstorms

- Individual is very open and impressionable; very **sensitive to pain and suffering of others**

- Worse from lying on **left side** of body

- Better with **reassurance** and **company**

OTHER HOME REMEDIES

Rescue Remedy

Rescue Remedy is a blend of five Bach flower remedies that can be used as emotional support in times of anxiety. It helps to reduce feelings of panic and anticipatory tension and can help to restore calm and focus.

Put four drops of Rescue Remedy directly on the tongue or add four drops to water and sip at intervals. Repeat as necessary.

Chamomile tea

This simple herbal tea is excellent for calming the nervous system and helping to promote relaxation. It's particularly helpful when anxiety causes sleep disturbance and is best taken in the evening before bed to encourage a good, restful night's sleep.

ATHLETE'S FOOT

A common fungal condition that appears on the feet and mostly affects the area between the toes. It can be recurring.

Signs of athlete's foot include:

- Very itchy and sore skin between the toes
- Cracking of the skin, especially between the toes
- Skin discoloration; may look darker in colour or red
- White flaky skin
- Small blisters filled with fluid on the surrounding skin
- Contagious; can spread to the soles, sides of the feet or toenails, causing a fungal nail infection

Actions that may help:

- Dry in between the toes after washing or when wet.
- Dab the feet gently when drying the affected area.
- Use a separate towel and washcloth.
- Wear cotton socks and change them daily.

- Uncover the feet, remove shoes and wear open-toed shoes and slippers.

You should seek medical advice if the foot shows signs of bacterial infection, such as becoming hot, painful and red, is foul smelling or very swollen.

Be careful when using products like antiperspirants to suppress sweat – use a natural deodorant. Sweating is the body's way of getting rid of things it needs to. By suppressing it, you're blocking your body's way of detoxing, driving the issue inwards.

HOMEOPATHIC REMEDIES

Baryta Carb

- **Cold** and **clammy** feet; **very smelly foot sweats**; toes and soles painful when walking; soles feel **hot** and **bruised** at night; sensitive to the cold; intolerable **itching** with burning and stinging; **needle-like pricking sensation**

- Often affects shy, **young children** who lack confidence, frequently have **swollen tonsils** and are slow to develop; and **elderly people** with confusion and **mental weakness**, who display child-like behaviour

- Worse at **night**; after **cold exposure** to the feet; from **suppressed foot sweat**

- Better for walking in **open air**

Graphites

- Moist, **thick, crusty eruptions** between toes that are **slow to heal**; cracks in between toes; thin, sticky, oozing **discharge**; **foul, acrid foot sweat** and **toe chafing**; **deformed**, thickened, cracked or **split toenails**; **inflamed nail root** with pus and infection; **cold feet**

- Worse from **heat**; **scratching**; in the **evening**

- Better in **open air**

Nitric-ac

- Profuse, **offensive foot sweat**; **soreness** of the toes; **cracks** and fissures between toes which crust and bleed easily; irritated, dry skin; very **sensitive to touch**; distorted, **discoloured**, yellow and curved toenails; **feet feel red and hot**, as though frozen; feeling like **walking on pins**; **splinter-like pains** under toenails; **irritable; pessimistic**

- Worse from **dampness; cold air**

- Better in **mild weather**

Silica

- Foot sweats with foul, **penetrating, rotting odour; corrosive sweat** that destroys socks and shoes; **ice-cold** and **sweaty** feet; sore soles; yellow, **brittle, split** and weak toenails

- **Fungal infections** are common as a result of excess sweating

- Worse with **suppressed foot perspiration**

- Better for **warmth** (clothing, heating, baths)

Thuja

- Strong, **sweet foot odour** (like garlic); **dry skin**, very sensitive to the touch (**needle-pricking sensation**); eruptions with **violent itching** or **burning**; inflamed toe tips; brittle, **ribbed**, soft, **discoloured** and **crumbling toenails**

- Feet can feel fragile, as if made from **wood or glass** (like they could break easily)

- Worse from **scratching**; **dampness**; **cold water**

- Better for **warmth**

Thuja is a good option for any fungal complaint.

OTHER HOME REMEDIES

Calendula herbal tincture or cream

Dilute the tincture in warm water to promote healing, reduce inflammation, clear up the infection and stop it from spreading. This is a good herbal tincture to include in a first aid box.

Add 10–15 drops to a small glass of warm, boiled (sterile) water for washing and cleaning. Reduce the number of drops if stinging occurs.

Apply Calendula cream twice daily if the skin is cracked and sore between the toes.

Apple cider vinegar foot bath

Mix one part apple cider vinegar with two parts warm water. Take daily foot baths until the symptoms improve. If the skin becomes irritated, dilute further by adding more water, or reduce the number of foot baths to once or twice a week.

Tea tree oil

If applying directly to the skin, dilute first by adding a few drops to a carrier oil (such as almond, coconut or olive oil), then dab gently onto the affected area. Add tea tree oil to a daily foot bath and soak for 15–20 minutes.

Garlic

Fresh garlic can be crushed or sliced and placed between the toes that have affected skin.

Bicarbonate of soda

Dust the inside of your shoes with bicarbonate of soda to absorb sweat and moisture, preventing the fungus from spreading.

BITES AND STINGS

Generally, a bite occurs when an insect uses its mouth to break through human skin, while a sting happens when an insect uses another body part, such as a stinger at its tail end, to pierce the skin and inject venom.

Signs of a bite or sting include:

- Redness in the affected area
- Swelling around the bite or sting
- Stinging or burning pain

Actions that may help:

- If visible, remove the stinger from an insect sting with care.
- Clean the area with warm water.
- Apply a cold, wet cloth or ice pack for 10 minutes to reduce or prevent swelling.
- Try not to damage the skin further by scratching the area.

When to seek medical advice:

- The bite or sting hasn't improved after a few days, or the site looks worse.

- The bite or sting is on the mouth, throat or close to the eyes.

- The affected area swells significantly (10cm or more around the site).

- There are signs of infection, such as increasing intensity of pain and heat, redness, swelling or pus.

- You develop a high fever, swollen lymph nodes or flu-like symptoms.

Go to A&E if you experience signs of a severe allergic reaction, including shortness of breath; a tight, constricted feeling in your chest; wheezing; swelling of the face, mouth or throat; and a sensation of constriction in your throat with difficulty swallowing.

HOMEOPATHIC REMEDIES

Apis Mel

- Affected part **red**, **hot**, **swollen**, sore, highly **sensitive to touch**; sting site looks **stretched** and **shiny**; **restlessness**; sudden sharp, **stinging** and **burning** pain

- Rapid **swelling**, especially after bee or insect stings

- Better for **cool applications**, e.g. ice

- Worse with **heat**; **touch**

If you try Apis Mel and no improvement
occurs, try Urtica Urens instead.

Belladonna

- **Hot, dry, throbbing, burning** skin; sudden, **rapid swelling** and **bright redness**; inflamed; very sensitive to **touch**; sharp, **stabbing pains**

- Worse from **jarring motion**; touch; **heat**; at **night**

- Better for **sitting**; being semi-erect

Cantharis

- Extremely painful with a strong **burning** sensation and **sharp** pains; very **irritated**; **obsessed** with **itching** the bite/sting site

- **Blister** formation and burning from bee stings

- Worse with **touch**; **heat**

- Better for **cold** application; **rubbing**

Cantharis is good for horsefly bites.

Hypericum

- More **tender** than the appearance would indicate; **hard, dry, yellow crusts** form on healing wound; **sharp, radiating pain**, especially in **nerve-rich areas**, e.g. fingertips, lips, soles of feet

- Insect stings or animal bites with a **puncture wound**; **lacerated** wounds (where there is tearing of the flesh)

- Worse from **touch**; **pressure**

- Better from **rubbing** the affected area

Ledum

- Discoloration of the affected area, looks **purple** and **puffy**; wound feels **cold to the touch**; desire for ice or very cold applications

- Protects or prevents bites and stings

- Worse with **warm applications**; heat

- Better for **cold applications**, e.g. bag of frozen vegetables

Ledum is the number one remedy for any puncture wounds from insect and animal bites or stings.

Urtica Urens

- **Itching**, **raised**, **red** blotches; burning heat with a **nettle rash**; burning and **stinging** pains

- Urticaria (hives) can affect the whole body

- Bites with **skin sensitivity**, e.g. flea bites

- Worse with **cool** applications; at **night**; with **water**; touch

- Better for **rubbing**

Urtica Urens may be used externally as a cream.

OTHER HOME REMEDIES

Bicarbonate of soda

This multiuse salt is a popular traditional home remedy found in most kitchens. It can help to reduce the pain and swelling from bee stings or insect bites. Mix a small amount of water with some bicarbonate of soda to make a thick paste, then apply it to the affected area. Leave it on for 15 minutes.

Calendula tincture or cream

Calendula soothes the affected skin and reduces soreness. Add a few drops of Calendula tincture to cooled boiled water or a saline solution to clean the site and reduce infection. Calendula cream can be applied to sore, tender skin.

Black tea

The tannic acid in black tea can reduce the itching, stinging pain and swelling of a sting or insect bite. Using warm water, wet a tea bag and apply it directly to the affected area.

Apple cider vinegar

This 'cure all' tonic is a recommended home remedy for many health problems due to its antimicrobial and antioxidant effects. Soak a cotton wool pad with apple cider vinegar and apply it to the bite to help reduce stinging and itching.

BUMPS AND BRUISES

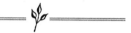

A bruise occurs after a blow or bump breaks the walls of localized blood vessels without breaking the skin. This causes blood to pool under the skin, leading to discoloration. The bruise will disappear as the body reabsorbs the blood during healing.

Signs of a bump or bruise include:

- Discoloration of the skin: red, purple, black, blue, brown or yellow

- Tenderness and pain at the site of the bump or bruise

- Swelling in the affected area

Actions that may help:

- Keep the area elevated and still; if moving it is painful, reduce any weight on the injury.

- Using an ice pack can have a numbing effect and help reduce swelling. For a homemade ice pack, wrap a cloth around a packet of frozen vegetables.

- Elevating the injured part to above the heart level can slow bleeding, reduce bruising, and prevent excessive swelling.

Seek medical help if there is a lot of bleeding, pain or excessive swelling. Get further advice if the swelling and pain don't start to reduce after a few days.

HOMEOPATHIC REMEDIES

Arnica

- **Sore**, uncomfortable and **fidgety**; may complain the **bed is too hard** and/or uncomfortable; damage to **muscles** and **soft tissues**

- Go-to remedy for **shock** or **trauma** following an injury; take **before or after surgery**, dental work or labour (mother and baby) to prevent trauma (emotional and physical) and bruising

- Worse for **touch**; **pressure**; **cold**; **motion**

- Better for **rest**; **lying down**

Arnica is recommended for most injuries and reduces swelling, relieves pain and prevents bruising.

Arnica cream

Arnica can also be used as a topical cream with immediate application for muscular pain, stiffness, sprains, bruises and minor injuries. Apply sparingly to the affected area with gentle massage three to four times daily.

Arnica cream should not be applied to broken skin.

Bellis Perennis

- Feeling of **bruising over whole body** after blows, falls, accidents, surgery; sore, bruised feeling in **pelvic region** after childbirth; trauma to **soft tissues**; **muscular soreness**, bruised and aching feeling

- First remedy for injury to **deeper tissues**; good for deep trauma and injuries to the **abdominal organs**

- Worse from **touch**; **cold baths**

- Better from **movement**; **pressure**; **heat**

Hypericum

- Sharp **shooting, radiating pain** upwards from injured part; feels as if **touched by an icy hand**

- Best for blows, bruising or crushing to **nerve-rich areas**; injuries to the **fingertips, toes** and **nails**; injuries to the **spine** or **genitals** and from bruising or displacement of the coccyx; **nerve pain** after dental work, e.g. root canals; **whiplash** and head injury

- Worse from **touch**; **pressure**; **jarring motion**

- Better from **sitting down**; **bending head back**; **rubbing** the sore spot

Ledum

- Very painful bruises, **sore** and **achy**; bruised area **feels cold**; bruised or **bloodshot eye**; **pressure** behind eyeballs; long-term bruising and **skin discoloration**

- After **puncture wound**, e.g. vaccination, blood test, IV, dental work; blows to the eye and for **black eyes**
- Worse with **motion**; **heat**
- Better for **cold applications**, e.g. ice pack

Ruta Grav

- Sore bruised **bone pain** with **aching**, **lameness**, **restlessness**; sharp, **shooting** pains and **stiffness**
- Injuries close to the bone; injuries to the **fibrous tissues** (tendons, ligaments and connective tissue); injuries to **back** and backache; twisting injuries to the **spine** and wrenching injuries, e.g. **shin bone**
- Worse from **overexertion**; cold; damp; **sitting**; lying on affected area
- Better for warmth or **heat**; **gentle motion**; and rubbing

Sul-ac

- Extensive bruising where the bruise turns **black** or **very dark blue**; deep or **persistent** bruise; **easy bruising** after slight bump
- Bruising from **injuries** or **surgery**; bleeding inside the **eyeball** after injury
- Worse from **pressure**; touch; the **cold**
- Better for **warmth**; lying on the affected side

Symphytum

- **Prickling pain** and soreness of the bone covering; **radiating pain** across the whole eyeball; **aching** pain

- Go-to for fractures and broken bones; good for blows and injuries from blunt instruments to **bone close to the skin** (face, shin, back of hands); injury and bruising of the **testicles**; blows and injury to the **eyeball**, black eyes; injuries to **coccyx**

- Worse with **touch**; **pressure**

- Better with **warmth**; **gentle motion**

> *Start with Arnica and then use*
> *Symphytum if symptoms persist.*

OTHER HOME REMEDIES

Rescue Remedy

Taken in times of stress, anxiety or shock, Rescue Remedy can be emotionally calming. Take four drops directly on the tongue or add four drops to water and sip at intervals. Repeat as necessary.

Essential oils

Lavender, tea tree and frankincense oils may help to speed up the skin's healing process by stimulating new cell formation. They also have antibacterial properties. These oils can be used separately or as a blend. Add a few drops to a carrier oil (such as almond, olive or coconut) and apply it to the affected area.

Parsley

Parsley is high in vitamin K, which stimulates blood clotting, reduces excessive bleeding and minimizes the extent of bruising.

Make a paste of fresh parsley leaves and a small amount of water, then apply directly to the bruised area. Cover with a dry gauze plaster to hold the paste in place.

Another option is to freeze the parsley paste into ice cubes and gently rub the bruise with the ice cube.

BURNS AND SCALDS

Burns are injuries to the skin caused by a heat source, exposure to a chemical or radiation. A scald is a burn caused by a hot liquid or steam. Burns are classified into four groups, based on the severity and extent of the damage:

- First-degree: redness of the skin; not blistered; skin is dry and intact

- Second-degree: blistered skin, moist and wet; blanches to pressure; very painful; can get worse over 24 hours

- Third-degree: deep burns with whiteness of the skin and thickened leathery appearance; skin doesn't blanche to pressure; hair comes away easily

- Fourth-degree: look like third-degree burns but other tissues are damaged, such as tendons or bone

Most first- and some second-degree burns can be treated at home if there is mild blistering and the skin is still intact.

Actions that may help:

- Run the affected part under lukewarm or cool water for five minutes to reduce the heat and burning pain.

- Keep the skin clean and resist breaking any blisters that form.

- Avoid interfering too much with the new healing skin; be gentle, and don't drag the skin or rub it.

Any burns with whiteness, charring, large blisters and that cover a large area (bigger than the palm of your hand) should be examined at A&E. Chemical burns also need immediate medical attention. The severity isn't determined by the level of pain; some deeper burns can be pain free.

HOMEOPATHIC REMEDIES

Arsenicum Album

- Burns with marked pain; **anxiety**; **restlessness**; feels **very chilly**; **exhaustion**; thirsty for **small sips of water**; **red**, burning, **swollen** skin, very **sensitive to the touch**

- Worse for **cold applications**; around **midnight**; with touch

- Better with **warm**, **dry applications**

Belladonna

- Sunburn with **dry**, hot and **bright red skin**; **radiates heat**; **craves lemons** or lemonade; **thirsty** for cold water; burning and **throbbing** pain; **pulsating headache** from excess sun exposure

- Worse with touch; **jarring motion**; **heat**

- Better for **rest**

Cantharis

- **Severe** sunburn; **intense, rapid** and extremely painful; **red, hot** skin; **blistering; swelling**; cutting, **stinging, raw, burning** pain

- Worse for **touch; movement**

- Better for **cold applications**, but once removed **pain starts again**

*Cantharis is the most common remedy
used for scalds and burns.*

Sol

- **Itching**; red, **blotchy** skin; painful **eyes**; photophobia; **blurry vision; headache; sensitive scalp**

- Sunstroke or sunburn; **radiation** burns; for people **sensitive to sunlight** who easily burn; can be used before going into strong sun

- Worse with **sunlight**

- Better from **pressure**; cold applications; short **naps**

Urtica Urens

- **Shiny** sunburn; intense **itching**; redness or **raised red blotches** (but no blistering); **burning** and **stinging** pain

- Simple scalds from **steam** or hot water

- Worse with **touch**; cool water; **bathing**; movement; after **sleep**

- Better when **lying down**

Similar to Cantharis, Urtica Urens can be used in a cream or gel and, when combined with Calendula, can be very soothing.

Phosphorus

When electrical burns occur, the damaged area may look small on the surface, but be more extensive underneath. A healthcare practitioner should always be consulted. On the way to seeking medical care, phosphorus can be used.

OTHER HOME REMEDIES

Topical application to burns or scalds

Apply sterile dressings soaked in a Hypericum or Hypericum and Calendula (Hyper Cal) solution made from 5ml (20 drops) of tincture in 200ml of cooled boiled water. Keep the dressing moist and disturb it as little as possible, re-dressing it every 12 hours until the skin is healed. Calendula ointment can be applied around the edge of the dressing.

Calendula

Calendula promotes skin healing, reduces inflammation and can stop infections from developing. To bathe the wound, add 10–15 drops of herbal tincture to cooled boiled water or a saline solution. If it stings, it can be further diluted.

Aloe vera

Also known as the 'burn plant', the gel found inside the leaf of the aloe vera plant has a cooling, healing effect. It's commonly used for minor burns, especially sunburn. To extract the gel, select a thick, large leaf and cut it at the base, allowing any yellow sap to drain away (as this can irritate the skin). Then, cut the leaf open and spoon out the clear, thick gel. Apply the gel to the burn using a dry, clean, non-sticky pad. If using a dressing or bandage, be careful to choose a pad that won't tear the skin when removing it.

Honey

Honey has natural antimicrobial and anti-inflammatory properties. It has been used as a remedy for thousands of years, dating back to Egyptian times. It can help reduce stinging pain and blistering in minor burns and is particularly effective for burns caused by oil splashes or scalds. To use, apply a thin layer to the burn and cover with a dressing if it's messy.

CHILBLAINS

Chilblains are small, irritating swellings on the skin that happen in response to cold temperatures. They typically develop several hours after exposure to the cold and heal on their own within two to three weeks. Chilblains commonly affect the fingers and toes, although they can also appear on the face.

Signs of chilblains include:

- Itching
- Burning sensation
- Discoloration of the skin, turning to red or purple
- Swelling

Actions that may help:

- Avoid going outside if it's cold.
- If hands or feet are cold, warm them up slowly.
- Wear gloves and thick woollen or cotton socks.
- Avoid itching or scratching chilblains as this can damage the skin.

HOMEOPATHIC REMEDIES

Agaricus

- **Redness** and swelling; **burning** and **itching**; cold, **numbness** and **tingling**; feet and toes can feel like they're **frozen**; feels very chilly; sensation as if pierced by **needles of ice** or **hot needles**; **creeping, crawling** sensation like ants on skin

- Chilblains of the face, nose, ears, toes and feet

- **Itching changes places** when scratched, followed by a burning sensation

- Worse with touch; cold, freezing air; **heat**

- Better with **slow walking**; when **warm in bed**

Petroleum

- Itching chilblains with **chapped, dry hands and feet**; **purple, stinging, hot** and **red feet** 'burn'; tips of fingers and skin between toes **crack and bleed easily from itching**; **moist, acrid-smelling discharge** from cracks

- Feet and hands can be cold and then go hot and itchy; parts can go cold after itching

- Worse in **cold weather**; when **itching** from the warmth in bed; from **dampness**

- Better in **dry, warm air**

Pulsatilla

- Hands, fingers, feet and toes are **hot**, red and **inflamed**; **coldness** and **numbness** of hands and feet; **inclination to stretch** the feet and toes; chilly; **thirstless**; weepy; **burning, itching,** swelling and pain in the hands and fingers

- Worse with **wet feet**; scratching; when hot (itching increases); when chilled; in the **evening**; in **bed**

- Better with **rubbing**; cold compress; in open air; from **walking**

Rhus Tox

- **Dark red**, inflamed skin; **smooth**, shiny skin; **swollen**, hot skin; restlessness; **crawling sensation** in fingertips; **tingling** feet; **intense itching** with burning and stinging after **scratching**

- Symptoms can be on the **left side** or go from **left to right**

- Worse from **getting wet**; when **cold** or chilled; skin is aggravated by cold, **open air**

- Better for **heat**; hot water; **warm compress**

OTHER HOME REMEDIES

Calendula tincture and cream

Calendula regenerates new skin cells, promotes healing and reduces inflammation. Use as a herbal tincture, warmed rather than cool, and dilute by adding 10–15 drops in water. Apply the tincture to the chilblains with a cotton wool pad or add to a foot bath.

Apply Calendula cream and massage twice daily to help with good blood circulation.

Thyme and ginger

To soothe chilblains using natural ingredients, add crushed ginger and thyme to a bowl of warm water and soak hands and feet.

Fill a large bowl with warm water to cover the feet. Take approximately seven fresh thyme sprigs or a few drops of thyme essential oil and add them to the bath. Grate the ginger and place it in a piece of stocking to keep it contained before adding it to the water.

Before dipping chilblained hands or feet directly into warm water, make sure to move them around actively to stimulate blood circulation. Avoid using hot water to prevent shock, especially if extremities are very cold or numb.

Onion and salt poultice

To create a soothing poultice for chilblains, begin by selecting enough onion to cover the affected area adequately. Mash the onion into a pulp using a mortar and pestle, then blend with a pinch of salt. Apply this blend with care to the inflamed skin, making sure the skin is intact and not open. Allow this natural remedy to sit for 15–20 minutes before washing it off. For additional relief, follow up with a gentle application of aloe vera gel to the area.

COLDS

Colds are common illnesses characterized by various symptoms that develop gradually over a few days. They tend to be milder than other respiratory illnesses, such as the flu. Most colds resolve on their own within a week or two without specific treatment. While adults and children can catch colds, symptoms tend to last longer in children.

Signs of colds include:

- Itchy, scratchy feeling in the back of the throat

- Sore throat

- Stuffy nose or runny nose: can alternate between the two

- Persistent sneezing or coughing

- Slight fever

- Headache, due to sinus pressure

- Fatigue

- Loss of smell and taste

Actions that may help:

- Rest and sleep.

- Drink plenty of fluids, including water and warm drinks.

- Steam inhalation helps with nasal congestion and irritated sinuses.

HOMEOPATHIC REMEDIES

Aconite

- **Sudden onset**; very first signs of a cold; sudden chill, **shivering**, fever; pain at **bridge of nose**; **dry**, congested, runny nose; **sneezing**; **anxiety**; physical and mental **restlessness**; very **thirsty** for large quantities of cold water

- Colds from exposure to **dry, cold winds**; getting very cold; or a **shock** or **fright**

- Worse in the **evening**; when **rising** from a lying position; at **midnight**

- Better in **open air**

Allium Cepa

- Predominantly affects **left side** of nose; profuse **watery, bland** nasal discharge; **prolific sneezing**; **acrid** nasal discharge that **drips** and burns; nose feels **raw**; red, burning eyes, **sensitive to light**; watery profuse tears; head feels dull and bunged up

- Springtime colds; colds caused by cold, damp weather or wet feet

- Worse from entering a **warm room** (causes sneezing); during the **evening**; in **spring**

- Better in cool, **open air**

Arsenicum Album

- Streaming from **right side** of nose and eyes; **thin, watery, acrid, burning nasal discharge**; **sore** and **chapped** nose; **bunged up** and itchy nose; **sneezing on waking** in the morning; **tired** and **weak**; **restlessness**; feels very chilly; thirsty for sips of water; **very fearful**; **desperate for company**

- Colds that go to the **chest**

- Worse in **cold, open air**; around **midnight** (between 11 p.m. and 2 a.m.)

- Better **indoors**; from **sitting up**; with **heat**

Euphrasia

- Streaming from the eyes and nose; profuse **watery eyes**; sensation of **sand in eyes**; irritation under eyelids; **stinging, acrid tears**; bland nasal discharge; constant **rubbing** of eyes or **blinking**; bloodshot eyes; **pain and pressure across forehead**; runny nose **during the day** but blocked up **at night**

- Colds that affect the **eyes**

- Worse during the **evening**; in **sunlight**; with **warmth**; in **wind**

- Better in **open air**; from **wiping eyes**; blinking; lying down; in **darkness**

Ferrum Phos

- **Slow onset** over a few days; beginning stages of cold; inflammation; red, **flushed** skin; **weary** and **lethargic**; watery nasal **discharge**; **thirsty** for cold water; **cold hands and feet**

- Individual may have a tendency to catch colds that often go to the **chest** and may get **nosebleeds** from cold temperatures

- Worse between **4 a.m. and 6 a.m.**; from **cold air**; **jarring motion**; **noise**

- Better from **gentle motion**; lying down; **rest**

Gelsemium

- **Gradual onset**; sensation of **heaviness** throughout the body; **drooping eyelids**; **fatigue, aching, weakness** and **soreness** of the body; **chills** up and down the back; congestion; irritating watery nasal discharge that feels like **hot water** flowing from the nose; **exhaustion** from **constant sneezin**g; thirstless; **dull headache**

- Typical flu or spring and summer colds

- Worse from cold; **damp** weather; **anticipation** (even of pleasurable events); **change in weather** (cold nights, warm days); from receiving bad news

- Better from **sweating**; **urination**; after **midday**; from being in **open air**

Natrum Mur

- **Violent sneezing**, especially early in the **morning** and in **sunlight**; streaming nose and watery eyes; watery or **egg-white nasal discharge**; loss of **smell** and **taste**; difficulty breathing; **sinusitis** with postnasal drip; sores and **ulcers inside the nose**; fever blisters on sides of nose; thirsty; desires **salty** things; blinding **headaches** with heaviness or bursting pain; **irritable**

- Can be caused by feelings of **grief** or **disappointment**

- Worse with a **cold wind**; sunlight; when **emotional**; on the seashore; between 9 a.m. and 11 a.m.
- Better in **open air**

Nux Vomica

- Fluent discharge of nose on **rising from bed**; **violent sneezing**; **nose runs when indoors** and during the daytime, **stuffed up** when **outdoors** and at night; blocked nose on **one side**; **hypersensitive** and **irritated** by everything; **very chilly** and shivery
- **Stuffy colds**; colds from exposure to cold, dry air; or **newborn snuffles**
- Worse in the **morning** on waking; when **cold**; in **open air**; with draughts; **air conditioning**; noise; lights
- Better with **rest**; **warmth**; after **eating**

OTHER HOME REMEDIES

Honey and lemon tea

Honey is known for its antimicrobial properties, while lemon provides a boost of vitamin C. Mix a tablespoon of honey and the juice of half a lemon in a cup of warm water. This mixture can soothe a sore throat and aid in the relief of cold symptoms.

Ginger tea

Ginger has anti-inflammatory properties and can help alleviate cold symptoms. Boil slices of fresh ginger root in water for a few minutes, then strain and drink the tea.

You can add lemon and honey to the tea for sweetness and additional benefits. Lemon acts as a natural detoxifier, helps in digestion and is rich in vitamin C, which can boost the immune system. Honey has antimicrobial properties that can help soothe a sore throat and other cold symptoms and fight infections.

Turmeric 'golden milk'

Curcumin, the key component of turmeric, boasts antiviral, antibacterial, and anti-inflammatory qualities. For centuries, this vibrant yellow spice has been a cornerstone in Ayurvedic medicine, especially for treating respiratory conditions.

Stir ¼ teaspoon of turmeric, a pinch of black pepper and a drizzle of ghee or sesame oil into a glass of warm milk and consume at bedtime.

COLD SORES

Cold sores are caused by the herpes simplex virus and are characterized by a crop of small blisters or dry, chapped eruptions that appear on the lips or around the nose. They can recur and outbreaks can be triggered by cold winds, changing hormones, stress, lowered immunity or the beginning of a cold. They usually clear up by themselves within 7–10 days.

Signs of cold sores include:

- Itchy, tingling sensation

- Soreness or burning

- Small fluid-filled blisters

Actions that may help:

- Avoid direct contact with someone who has a cold sore, as they are contagious.

- Don't share lip balm or use the same utensils as someone with a cold sore.

- Use lip balm to protect the lips from cold or hot weather.

- Reduce stress, as this can trigger cold sores.

HOMEOPATHIC REMEDIES

Graphites

- **Moist**, **crusty** eruptions around the mouth and nose, especially in the corners; **oozing honey-like** discharge; **itching** and **burning** blisters, slow to heal

- Worse from **heat**; at **night**

- Better in **open air**

Natrum Mur

- Cold sores around mouth or lips; **dry** and **cracked** lips and corners of mouth; **tingling** in lips; desires **salty food**; **thirsty** for large quantities of water

- Can appear after an emotional upset – a **grief**, **loss** or **disappointment** – or in people that don't like to express their emotions and often keep them in

- Worse in **sunlight**; from sun exposure; **suppressed emotions**; at the seashore

- Better in **open air**

Rhus Tox

- **Yellow blistering** around the mouth or lips; neuralgic **shingle-like pains**; itching; burning

- Worse in **cold**, **damp** weather; from being chilled

- Better for **heat**; warm applications

Sepia

- **Exhaustion**; no energy; **very irritable**; wants to be left alone
- For cold sores that arise around **menstruation, pregnancy, childbirth** and **menopause**
- Worse from **cold air**; **hormonal changes**
- Better for **hot applications**

OTHER HOME REMEDIES

Tea tree oil

As an antiviral, tea tree oil can prevent cold sores. Apply at the first sign of tingling to resolve an outbreak. Dilute the oil by adding a few drops to a carrier oil (such as almond, coconut or olive oil), then dab it onto the cold sore intermittently throughout the day.

Lemon balm

Another antiviral, lemon balm can be applied to reduce the redness and irritation from a cold sore and help to dry it up.

COLIC

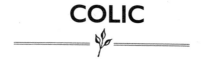

Colic appears in young babies and presents with excessive screaming for hours, which can't be relieved by their caregivers. It usually appears around six weeks of age and stops at 3–4 months. Colic usually gets worse in the evening.

Signs of colic include:

- Gastric discomfort

- Gas and bloating, belly is tight

- Distress, crying, screaming with a red face

- Clenched fist

- Writhing around

- Raising legs up

- Inconsolable

Actions that may help:

- Rock baby or massage their tummy or back.

- Cuddle baby, then hold them close.

- Put baby into a warm bath to help calm and relax.

If the colic doesn't seem to be getting better and nothing seems to work, contact your healthcare practitioner. You can also seek help for support and guidance on coping strategies.

HOMEOPATHIC REMEDIES

Aethusa

- Baby unable to **hold the weight** of their own head; **muscular weakness**; **very hungry** but never satisfied; frequently regurgitates then wants to feed again; **projectile vomiting** of large curds after being fed; **weakness** after vomiting; great distress, crying a lot and squirming; **clenched thumbs**, eyes turn downwards, **red face**; unsettled, **disturbed sleep**; appears **sad** rather than angry

- A good remedy for babies with a **milk intolerance** (either breast milk or formula)

- Worse after **drinking milk**; from **vomiting**

- Better in **open air**

Chamomilla

- Hot tummy, **swollen with wind**; loose, smelly, **grass-green stools** (like chopped eggs and spinach); **angry**; screaming and shrieking; **legs drawn up** to the tummy; crying; **restlessness**; **sleeplessness**

- Worse for **touch**; between **9 p.m. and midnight**; from **heat**

- Better for **being carried** on the shoulder; **fast rocking**; with **cold compress**

Chamomilla is one of the most common remedies for colic in babies.

Colocynthis

- Unbearable **cutting, griping pain**, comes in waves; post-feed colic; sour, **jelly-like stools**; angry; **extremely irritable**; pulls **knees up to chest**; wriggles, twists and turns with **distorted face**, restlessness; loud, cross crying

- Worse when **feeding**; with the slightest **touch**; at **4 p.m.**; when **lying on back**

- Better when **laid tummy-down or over the shoulder**; when **bending double** or pressing **something hard** against abdomen to get relief; from warmth; bending head forward; after defecating

Dioscorea

- Unbearable **sharp**, twisting, **griping pain**; excessive **wind**

- Worse from **bending forward**; **lying down**

- Better for bending, arching or **stretching backwards** to get relief; from **sitting upright**; moving about

Ipecac

- Hard to please; **never settles**; inconsolable; frantic; fist chewing; **frequently regurgitates** small amounts of milk after feeding; **stiffens out** during a paroxysm of pain, body is **straight** and **rigid**; **grass-green stools**, foamy with **white mucus**

- Worse from **over-feeding**; when breast-feeding mother eats rich foods; from **medication** given to mother during birth or after surgery

- Better with **pressure**

Ipecac is the remedy to use if pethidine was used during labour and the baby has colic.

Lycopodium

- Bloated abdomen; grunting and wriggling; **trapped wind**; baby seems **very hungry** but feels very full after eating very little; post-feed **bloating**

- Worse if breast-feeding mother eats **windy foods** such as cabbage and beans; in the evening between **4 p.m. and 8 p.m.**

- Better for **burping**; **passing wind**

Mag Phos

- Burping; **spasmodic** gut, intermittent waves of pain; **anxiety**; fearful; **restlessness**

- Worse at **night**; from **drinking milk**; from **touch**

- Better for **heat**; warmth; from **bending double**; with **abdominal massage**; with **pressure** on belly from lying on abdomen; with belly pressed against a shoulder

Nux Vomica

- **Constipation**; griping, cramping, painful **spasms**; frequent crying; baby draws feet up and kicks them out again in **anger** or arches backward; extreme **sensitivity** and **irritability**; cold hands and feet

- Worse when breast-feeding mother has a diet that's **too rich** or **stimulating**, e.g. spicy food, caffeine

- Better for **passing stool**; passing wind; **warmth**

OTHER HOME REMEDIES

Warm bath

A warm bath in the evening can be calming and help to relax tense muscles.

Gentle massage with oils

Special massage techniques can help babies with colic and aid digestion. They can be practised at home or at a local baby massage class. Add a few drops of essential oil – such as lavender, chamomile or peppermint – to a carrier oil, like olive oil. Warm the oil by rubbing your hands together, then gently massage baby's tummy clockwise.

Food choices

In rare cases, babies have intolerances as their digestion is very immature. Usually, the colic is accompanied by vomiting or happens after every feed rather than coming on in the evening. Review the mother's diet: try cutting out caffeine and spicy foods. If a sensitivity is suspected, cut out dairy or gluten for a few weeks, one food at a time, and seek further advice.

CONJUNCTIVITIS

Conjunctivitis (pink eye) is caused by inflammation of the membrane that covers the eyeball and under the lids. One or both eyes may be affected. Discharge is often thick and sticky.

The eyes may become red and sore due to a bacterial infection, resulting in a yellow, thick discharge. This can also be caused by an allergy or hay fever, leading to red, itchy and uncomfortable eyes.

Signs of conjunctivitis include:

- Whites of the eyes can be pink, red or bloodshot

- Eyes become sore and itchy, with a gritty feeling

- Burning sensation

- Yellow, thick, sticky discharge

Actions that may help:

- If it's an allergy or hay fever, try placing a cold, wet flannel over the eyes.

- If it's a bacterial infection, gently clean the eyes with cooled boiled water, to remove any discharge or crusts.

- Wash hands regularly and don't share face cloths to avoid bacterial transmission.

HOMEOPATHIC REMEDIES

Aconite

- **Sudden onset**; **beginning stages** of conjunctivitis; **dry**, **hot** feeling in the eye; sensation of **sand in eyes**; red, **bloodshot** and sore eyes; **red**, **swollen** eyelids; **anxiety**; restlessness

- Conjunctivitis after **injuries**, surgery, or a **foreign body** in the eye; or can start after being out in **dry**, **cold winds**

- Worse with **light**; **tobacco smoke**; at **night**

- Better in **open air**

Argent Nit

- **Swollen**, red, inflamed eyes, **sensitive to light**; smelly, **creamy**, **yellow discharge** glueing eyelids together; eyelids look like **raw beef**; aching, tired eyes, can't focus; **sugar cravings**; **anticipation** and **apprehension**

- Inflammation of eyes in **babies**

- Worse for being in a **warm room**; in **left eye**; from being **emotional**; from **wind** blowing on face

- Better for **cold compress**; **pressure**; closing eyes; cool air

Arsenicum Album

- Watery, burning, **inflamed**, hot eyelids; **corrosive tears**, makes cheeks and eyelids **sore**; eyes stick together with **crusts, stinging pain** on opening; intense **photophobia**; **restlessness**; anxiety about health and disease; thirsty for cold water but takes only **little sips**

- Worse in **sunlight**; around **midnight** (between 11 p.m. and 2 a.m.); lying on **right side**; when **cold**

- Better with **warm compress**; with **company**; when **sitting up**; elevating the head; in **open air**

Euphrasia

- Hot, burning, **streaming** tears; constantly **wiping/rubbing eyes** or **winking**; thick, sticky, **yellow, acrid mucus** in the corners of eyes; sensation of **sand in eyelids**; swollen, burning eyelids; **bland nasal discharge**; **sharp pain** from bright light

- Conjunctivitis with **measles**

- Worse when **warm**; in the **evening**; with **sunlight**; from **wind** exposure

- Better in **open air**; from **blinking**; lying down; in **darkness**

Pulsatilla

- **Thick**, profuse, bland, **yellow (green) discharge** with sticking of the eyelids; eyelids inflamed and stuck together (but not painful); itching, burning eyes; **rubbing eyes**; weepy and **emotional**; thirstless

- **Neonatal** conjunctivitis in very young babies; or conjunctivitis from **a cold** or from **measles**
- Worse in a stuffy, **warm room**; on **waking**; at **twilight**
- Better for company and **sympathy**; **crying**; **motion**; in **open air**

OTHER HOME REMEDIES

Euphrasia tincture

Euphrasia, also known as eyebright, is useful as a tincture to relieve and clear the infection. Add 10 drops of Euphrasia tincture to ½ pint (approximately 300ml) of cooled boiled water and mix in a teaspoon of salt. Using a cotton pad or clean cloth, bathe the eyes 3–4 times daily.

Chamomile tea soak

Chamomile has natural soothing properties that can help reduce inflammation and irritation. Brew a cup of chamomile tea, then cool to a comfortable temperature. Soak a clean cloth or cotton pad in the tea then use as a compress on the closed eye.

CONSTIPATION

An individual who passes fewer than three bowel movements in a week, with stools that are large, hard or lumpy, may be experiencing constipation. Typically, a person with a healthy digestive system will have one bowel movement daily. It's worth noting that constipation is quite common during pregnancy and can persist for several weeks postpartum. In rare cases, it may be indicative of an underlying medical condition.

Signs of constipation include:

- Pain or difficulty passing stools
- Infrequent bowel movements
- Large, hard stools
- Stomach ache
- Bloating
- Nausea

Actions that may help:

- Increase dietary fibre, which is found in fruits, vegetables and grains.

- Increase fluid intake in the diet.

- Take part in regular exercise and physical movement.

- Don't ignore the urge to go to the bathroom.

- Check out the side effects of conventional medications.

- Address any emotional stress, anxiety or depression.

HOMEOPATHIC REMEDIES

Alumina

- **Paralysis of the bowels**; great **straining**; no urge to defecate; hard, dry, **knotty stools**; sore, dry, **inflamed rectum**; might only be able to pass stool **standing up**; confusion; craves **dry food** and avoids liquids

- Obstinate, severe constipation in **babies**, **infants** or the **elderly** who haven't passed a stool in days

- Worse from drinking **formula milk**; eating **potatoes** and highly processed foods; in the **morning**

- Better from **moderate exercise**; at **night**; with **warm drinks**

Bryonia

- Large, **dry**, **hard**, **black stools**, painful to pass with great effort, can smell like **old cheese**; burning pain in anus during or after defecating; **thirsty** for cold drinks; **dry mouth**; cracked lips; **irritable**; **headaches**

- Constipation in **pregnancy** and in babies

- Worse with **motion**; in **hot weather**

- Better from **hard pressure**, e.g. massage or rubbing; from being **alone**

Calc Carb

- **Large, hard, pale stools**, chalk-like in appearance, **sour-smelling**; **prolapse** or **haemorrhoid** from straining; slow, **sluggish digestion**; **craves eggs and indigestible things** such as soil, chalk or coal

- Can be used for constipation that is **not uncomfortable** or painful, where the individual feels well; for **babies** and **infants** who **cry a lot** and **body movement** increases before passing a large stool

- Worse with **tight-fitting** clothes or bed coverings; with **hormonal changes**; from drinking **milk**

- Better for **passing gas**

Natrum Mur

- **Very dry stool**, hard and **crumbling**, coated with **glassy mucus**; **constriction of rectum** with **burning, tearing, itching** around the anus after defecating; **anal fissures, bleeding** and stinging; haemorrhoids; constipation on **alternate days**

- Individual is constipated when **away from home**, due to inability to use other toilets than their own; or constipation following **grief, loss** or **disappointed love**

- Worse from **strong emotions**

- Better in **open air**

Nux Vomica

- The stool is infrequent and difficult to pass, **lots of urging** with no result; passes a **small amount** of stool and **feels as if unfinished**; **angry**; impatient; **irritable**; oversensitive; **overactive mind**

- **Inactivity** and obstinate constipation after lots of **rich food**; overeating; taking too many **laxatives**

- Worse from the **cold**; noise; **tight clothing around the waist**

- Better for naps; **resting**; **warm drinks**

Sepia

- Large, **hard stools** covered with a **jelly-like mucus** that cannot be passed despite **straining**; sensation of **lump or ball in the rectum**; not able to empty bowels fully; very **irritable**; sensitive; **exhausted**; emotionally numb; **haemorrhoids in pregnancy**

- Often seen in **pregnancy** or around **menstruation**

- Worse from **hormonal changes**; after **eating**

- Better for **exercise**; **movement**

Silica

- Much urging but feels like rectum **doesn't have enough power** to pass the stool; **straining** with sweating, **weakness** and **exhaustion**; rectal pain; stool starts to come out but **goes back in again**; painful, **spasmodic constrictions** of anal sphincter muscle; **anal fissures**; **painful haemorrhoids**; lacks self-confidence; timid

- Constipation always **before and during menstruation**

- Worse from the **cold**; **draughts**

- Better for **warmth**

OTHER HOME REMEDIES

Black sesame seeds and walnuts

Take equal quantities of black sesame seeds and walnuts. Fry them in a pan or wok without using any oil until they are slightly toasted. Let them cool and then roughly crush them. Consume one heaped tablespoon of this mixture daily with half a pint of water. This method is meant to direct the water to the large intestine, stimulating bowel movement.

Organic golden linseed

Linseed (also known as flaxseed) is very rich in fibre and helps stimulate bowel movement. Break the shell of the seeds by grinding them in a pestle and mortar or coffee grinder, otherwise the body will pass them whole. The ground linseed can be sprinkled over food or added to a smoothie. It's also important to drink plenty of water whilst taking linseed.

Start with one tablespoon a day and increase to three tablespoons per day if required.

COUGHS

A cough is a natural reflex that helps to clear the airways of mucus or is the result of inflammation of the mucous membranes associated with a cold or flu virus. It can also result from inhaling external particles such as dust or smoke.

A cough is usually not indicative of a serious condition and most resolve on their own within three weeks without needing treatment. Consult your doctor for a persistent cough lasting a few weeks.

There are two main types of cough:

- Dry coughs, which are irritating and don't produce mucus (such as croup)

- Chesty coughs that produce mucus or phlegm

Other types of cough include:

- Dry, hacking coughs that lead to discomfort in the chest and sleep disturbance

- Spasmodic and repetitive coughs

Actions that may help:

- Drink plenty of fluids.

- Consume hot drinks containing lemon and honey.

- Rest, but avoid lying flat on your back.

HOMEOPATHIC REMEDIES

Aconite

- **First sign** of a cough; **sudden onset**; **high fever** or coldness with chills and **shivering**; **hoarse**, dry, barking, suffocating, **croupy** cough; **tickly** throat; very thirsty; **restlessness**; great **anxiety**, sense of **foreboding**

- Coughs from **shock**; getting very cold; exposure to **dry, cold winds**

- Worse at night (starts or gets worse around **midnight**); from drinking **cold water**

- Better from **open air**; **rest**

Ant Tart

- **Suffocating, rattly cough**; **very little mucus** coughed up; difficulty breathing; **phlegm on the chest**; vomiting of **thick, white, ropey mucus**; feeling of **drowning** or suffocation, **must sit up**; **exhausted** and **drowsy** after coughing fit; thirsty for cold water

- Children with frequent colds leading to **chesty coughs** with mucus

- Worse from being **looked at**; in warm, **stuffy rooms**; from **heat**; eating; **lying down**; **anger**; cold, **damp weather**; being touched

- Better for cool, **open air**; lying on **right side**; sitting up; **vomiting**; **coughing up** mucus; being left alone

Bryonia

- Slow, **gradual onset**; hard, **dry, hacking, painful** cough; **irritability of upper trachea** (windpipe); **holds chest to keep it still**; **soreness** with sharp, **stabbing pains** in sides of chest; **dry throat**, very little phlegm; **irritable**; very **thirsty**, drinks in large gulps; headaches

- Cough causes the individual to involuntarily leap from their bed or chair

- Worse from **movement**; talking; laughing; **entering a warm room**; inhaling; at night

- Better from **being still**; cool, **open air**; resting; lying on painful side; with **hard pressure**; having cold drinks

Drosera

- **Dry**, irritating, **spasmodic** cough; **rapid, continued** coughing; difficulty breathing; **retching** and **vomiting**; cough sounds **deep** and **hoarse, barking** or **choking**; **holds chest** when coughing; **tight** chest; **tickly throat**; yellow phlegm

- Cough starts as soon as the head hits the pillow and from the warmth of the bed

- Worse from **lying down**; **talking**; **after midnight**; in a stuffy room

- Better from **pressure**; **sitting up** in bed; **motion**; being quiet; in **open air**

Hepar Sulph

- Noisy, **hoarse**, **dry cough**; loose, **rattly** cough; **croupy, choking** cough; **thick yellow mucus**; **must stand up** to cough with **head bent back**; sensation of **fish bone/splinter** stuck in the throat; **very chilly**; extremely sensitive to the cold; **irritable**

- Coughs from exposure to dry, cold air, especially from west or northwest winds; or from exposure to a cold draught after getting **chilled**

- Worse from **cold air**; getting cold; walking; eating or drinking anything cold; in the **early morning**

- Better in a **warm room**; from wrapping up; with **heat**

Phosphorous

- Violent, hollow, **dry cough**; burning, dry, **tickly** throat; **hot feeling** in chest, behind breastbone; painful, throbbing head; difficulty sleeping; transparent or **blood-streaked phlegm**; **anxiety**; craves company and sympathy

- Coughs from **change in the weather**; windy, cold weather; getting wet in hot weather; or every cold leads to a **chesty cough**

- Worse at night; when moving from a **warm room into cold air**; lying on **left side**; from talking or laughing

- Better from touch; massage; **sitting up**; lying on **right side**; cold drinks

Pulsatilla

- **Changeable symptoms**, e.g. loose cough in the morning, dry in the evening; rattling cough; short, dry, hacking cough; **thick**, **yellow mucus**; runny nose; **tickling in upper abdomen**; headache; retching; **thirstless**; craves **affection** and **sympathy**; shyness; **weepy**, **clingy** and whingey

- Coughs from **abandonment**; grief; a **chill**; getting **wet feet**

- Worse at night (dry), morning (loose); from being **left alone**; in **warm**, **stuffy** rooms

- Better from cool, **fresh**, **open air**; cold drinks; **sitting up with head high**; rubbing and massage

Rumex Crispus

- Incessant, **dry**, **suffocating**, **tickling**, **exhausting** cough; tickly throat; breathlessness; **urinating when coughing**; persistent **sticky**, **white phlegm** in the larynx, difficult to cough up; **stringy mucus**

- Coughs from **changing temperatures**: cold to warm, warm to cold

- Worse from touching or pressing **pit of the throat**; **inhaling cold air**; **undressing**; **talking**; on waking in the morning; at **night** (up to 11 p.m.); lying on **left side**

- Better with **warmth**; from **wrapping up**; **covering mouth and head**

Spongia

- Harsh, **dry**, **barking**, **croupy** cough; '**foghorn**' sound; **burning** in throat, larynx and chest; soreness deep in chest; **dryness of all air passages**; feels like '**breathing through a sponge**'; cough sounds 'dry as a bone', like a saw being driven through pine board, or a seal's bark; choking on falling asleep; **anxiety**

- Worse from **talking**; dry, cold winds; exertion; cold drinks; lying on **right side**; when inhaling; **before midnight**

- Better with **eating** or **drinking** (especially warm drinks); sucking on sweets; **swallowing**; bending head forward

OTHER HOME REMEDIES

Steam inhalation

Ease coughing and congestion by inhaling steam, which can help moisten the airways and thin mucus. Fill a bowl with steaming, hot water, lean over it and use a towel to cover the head and trap the steam. Inhale for several minutes.

Eucalyptus oil

Adding a few drops of eucalyptus oil, which has natural decongestant properties, to a steam inhalation can help reduce coughing and clear up mucus. Moreover, putting a few drops of the oil on a pillow at night or on a tissue beside the bed can help with nighttime coughing.

Thyme

Thyme can significantly reduce coughing and is a natural decongestant. Add a few sprigs to a steam inhalation or make a tea by steeping the fresh herb in hot water for a few minutes.

Honey tea

Honey is well regarded for its soothing properties and its ability to provide relief from coughing.

Mix two teaspoons of honey with warm water or herbal tea. Drinking this mixture can help reduce coughing frequency and improve sleep quality, especially when a nighttime cough occurs.

Turmeric 'golden milk'

Curcumin, the key component of turmeric, boasts antiviral, antibacterial and anti-inflammatory qualities. For centuries, this vibrant yellow spice has been a cornerstone of Ayurvedic medicine, especially for treating respiratory conditions.

Stir ¼ teaspoon of turmeric, a pinch of black pepper and a drizzle of ghee or sesame oil into a glass of warm milk and drink at bedtime.

CUTS, GRAZES
AND WOUNDS

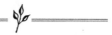

Types of cuts, grazes and wounds include:

- Abrasion: a graze or scrap involving the top layer of the skin

- Laceration: a deep cut or tear to the skin made by a sharp object

- Incision: usually refers to a surgical cut, a deep cut made by a knife

- Puncture wound: caused by a sharp, pointed object, such as a nail, creating a deep hole

Actions that may help:

- Wounds need to be kept clean to prevent infections developing. Clean the wound with cooled boiled water or saline solution.

- Puncture wounds need a good clean. Hold under running water for five minutes to flush out dirt, then clean the surrounding skin.

- Cover the injury with a dressing or plaster if it's bleeding or if the skin is torn.

- Once the area looks dry, it can be exposed to the air and form a scab.

- If there's a lot of bleeding, apply some pressure and elevate above the heart level. Clean once the bleeding has stopped.

Signs of an infected wound:

- Redness and swelling

- Wound site feels warm to the touch

- Constant pain or soreness

- Discharge of green or yellow pus

- Slow or poor healing

- Red streaks on the skin, coming from the wound

- Fever or chills

When to seek medical attention:

- Any deep wound with soft tissue exposed, such as tendons or bone, or a skin tear that will need to be held together by stitches to heal.

- If there are signs of infection such as smelly pus, redness, heat and swelling, or if it looks like it's getting worse.

HOMEOPATHIC REMEDIES

Arnica

- **Sore** and **bruised** feeling; fear of touch or being examined; individual claims to be OK, avoids attention, may be in **shock**

- Use after **traumatic injuries**, recent or in the past; before and after **surgery**; after **dental extraction**

- Worse from **touch**

- Better from **lying down**

DO NOT put Arnica cream on an open wound.

Calc Sulph

- Inflamed; with **oozing** thick, **yellow**, lumpy, **bloody pus**; **slow to heal**; unhealthy skin

- Worse with **touch**; the **cold**; in a **heated room**

- Better in **open air**; when **bathing**; with **heat**

Hepar Sulph

- Infection with **yellow, foul-smelling pus** (like **old cheese**); **throbbing, splinter-like** pain; redness; swelling; **tenderness**

- Worse in the **cold**; with **touch**

- Better for **heat**

Hypericum

- **Nerve-rich** areas; **sensitive** to touch; **sharp, shooting** pains from the wound; extremely painful

- Use for clean cuts from **surgery**; **lacerations**; **puncture** wounds; **crushed** fingers; after surgery/procedures affecting the **spine**, e.g. epidural

- Worse with **touch**; jarring motion; the **cold**

- Better from **rubbing**

Lachesis

- **Mottled** skin, **bluish**, **purplish** appearance; **infected** wound with burning pain; **hypersensitive** skin, intolerance to **touch** or **constriction**

- Use for puncture wounds; **animal bites**; small wounds that bleed significantly; bedsores; ulcers

- Worse with **tight-fitting clothes**; slight touch; heat

- Better for **warm applications**; with **loose clothes**

Ledum

- **Stinging** pain that travels upwards; wounded area feels **cold to touch**, looks **purple** and **puffy**; desires ice or very cold applications

- Use for **puncture** wounds from **animal bites**, injections, stepping on nails; splinters; **penetration** wounds, especially on hands or soles of feet

- Worse from **warm applications**; **covering affected area**; at **night**

- Better for **cold applications**

Nitric-ac

- Very painful, **slow healing** wounds; foul-smelling, dirty, green discharge; raw, bleeding ulcers; **splinter-like** pains; very sensitive; chilly; angry and **irritable**

- Worse with **touch**; **cold air**; **heat**; **jarring motion**

- Better for steady **pressure**

Staphysagria

- Intense pain after **cleaning** affected area; inflammation; feelings of **anger** and **humiliation**

- Use for inflamed **lacerations**, incisions, **stab** wounds; cuts from **sharp** instruments; for lingering pain after **surgery**; after **episiotomy** (incision to perineum); after **tooth extraction**

- Worse in the **cold**; with **touch**

- Better for **warmth**; **rest**

OTHER HOME REMEDIES

Calendula

Calendula possesses antifungal, anti-inflammatory and antibacterial properties, making it beneficial for healing cuts, grazes and wounds. It promotes healing, reduces inflammation and clears infection, so it's a valuable addition to your first aid kit.

Calendula tincture

Make sure the cut is clean and any debris has been removed. To clean wounds, add 10–15 drops of the tincture to a small glass of cooled boiled (or sterile) water. Dilute further if stinging occurs.

This tincture is useful after childbirth (tears or surgery), when used to wash the perineum.

Calendula tincture, diluted in water, can also be used as a mouthwash after dental work.

Calendula cream

Make sure the cut is clean and any debris has been removed, then apply a thin layer of cream to the affected area three times a day, or as needed.

Hypericum and Calendula cream (Hyper Cal)

Made from the natural herbal preparation of Calendula (Marigold) combined with Hypericum (St John's Wort), Hyper Cal can be used for cuts, abrasions, wounds, and stinging and cutting pains. It promotes rapid healing, provides pain relief and is an antiseptic.

Turmeric

Turmeric is rich in curcumin, which has been shown to have many healing effects. It's antibacterial, anti-inflammatory and antioxidant with remarkable wound-healing properties.

Mix ground turmeric with cooled boiled water to make a thick paste. Apply the paste to the wound and cover it with a bandage. Don't disturb it for 12–24 hours. After that, change the dressing and clean the wound. Repeat this process for three days to promote healing and prevent scarring.

Cayenne pepper

Cayenne pepper can be used to stem bleeding. Wash the wound using clean water, then sprinkle a small amount of ground cayenne pepper on the bleeding area. Elevate the area if possible. Once the bleeding has stopped, clean the area again thoroughly and cover it with a plaster or sterile dressing.

Witch hazel

Witch hazel can minimize bleeding. Its astringent effects reduce blood flow, promote clotting and constrict the blood vessels. To stop bleeding, apply witch hazel to gauze and press it against the wound. Use pure witch hazel; avoid products with alcohol or other additives.

CYSTITIS

Cystitis, also known as a urinary tract infection (UTI), is an acute bladder infection that is more common in women. It's often mild and can clear up on its own after a couple of days of drinking plenty of fluids. However, some people experience chronic recurrent cystitis and may require the advice of a qualified healthcare practitioner.

Signs of cystitis include:

- Burning, cutting or stinging pain

- Worse pain on passing urine or afterwards

- Urgency to pass urine more frequently than normal

- Passing urine in small amounts

- No relief on passing urine

- Urge to pass urine again soon after urination

- Cloudy, dark or foul-smelling urine

Actions that may help:

- Drink plenty of fluids.

- Avoid caffeinated or fizzy drinks.

- Wear cotton underwear and avoid tight-fitting jeans or leggings.

- Maintain good hygiene and wash regularly with unperfumed soaps.

- Don't delay urinating and always empty the bladder fully.

Seek immediate medical care if symptoms get worse and include high fever, pain that radiates down the back or sides and blood in the urine.

HOMEOPATHIC REMEDIES

Apis Mel

- **Burning** and **soreness** while urinating; **stinging, sharp** pain; **last drops of urine** burn and smart; urinating more than drinking; **thirstless**; constant desire to urinate, especially at night

- Worse with **heat**; pressure; **touch**; from lying down; between 4 p.m. and 5 p.m.

- Better from feeling cool; **cold applications**, e.g. flannel, compress, cold bath

Cantharis

- Intolerable, **constant desire** to urinate; violent, **cutting pain before, during and after urination**; **burning**, scalding urine; urine passed drop by drop; dreads going to the toilet; griping pain in bladder; burning thirst but aversion to drinking

- Worse from urinating; **sound of water**; drinking cold water; at **night**

- Better for **warmth**; lying down; with **quiet**

Nux Vomica

- Painful, **ineffectual urge** to urinate; **irritable bladder** from spasmodic sphincter; **not able to pass urine**; frequently going to the toilet, little and often; **itching in urethra** and **pain in neck of bladder** whilst urinating; **irritable** and **angry**

- Worse from **beer** or **wine**

- Better for **resting**; with **hot drinks**

Sarsaparilla

- Bladder feels **tender** with urge to urinate; severe **pain as urine ceases to flow**; **screaming** from pain; urine dribbles and **feeble flow**; **must stand** to urinate

- Worse when **sitting**

- Better when **standing**

Staphysagria

- **Pressure** on bladder; bladder **never feels fully empty**; frequent urging to urinate with scanty or profuse **watery urine**; sensation of **drop of urine rolling along urethra**; sits on toilet for long periods of time; **burning pain** in urethra **during and after urinating**

- **Honeymoon** cystitis, from new or frequent sex; cystitis after **surgery** or internal examination; cystitis caused by **humiliation, suppressed anger**, indignation

- Worse with anger; at **night**; after urination; **after sex**

- Better for **warmth**; **rest**

OTHER HOME REMEDIES

Thyme tea

Boil some water and add fresh or dried thyme. Brew for 15 minutes, strain and drink. The warmth of the tea can also provide some comfort and can be taken 2–3 times a day. Add honey to sweeten the tea if desired.

Bicarbonate of soda

Due to its alkaline properties, bicarbonate of soda can help ease the symptoms of cystitis. It makes the urine less acidic and alleviates the burning sensation. Mix one teaspoon of bicarbonate of soda with a glass of water and stir it until fully dissolved. Drink the mixture on an empty stomach or at least 20 minutes before meals.

DIARRHOEA

Diarrhoea is characterized by loose, watery stools passed frequently from the bowels. It can range from a mild, temporary condition to a potentially life-threatening one.

Causes of diarrhoea include infections by bacteria, viruses or parasites; consumption of contaminated food or water; certain medications; and diseases affecting the stomach, small intestine or colon.

Signs of diarrhoea include:

- Frequent watery stools

- Abdominal cramps

- Bloating

- Urgent need to use the bathroom

Actions that may help:

- Drink plenty of fluids.

- Avoid alcohol and caffeinated drinks.

- Follow the BRAT diet – bananas, rice, applesauce and toast

- Try an electrolyte replacement solution.

- Supplement with probiotics or eat foods rich in healthy bacteria such as kefir or live yogurt.

Severe cases of diarrhoea may lead to dehydration, which requires prompt medical attention, especially in young children and the elderly. Most cases of diarrhoea resolve on their own within a few days, but chronic or severe diarrhoea may require medical treatment.

HOMEOPATHIC REMEDIES

Argent Nit

- **Watery** stools, green like **chopped spinach**; noisy **flatulence**; bloating of abdomen; loud belching

- Diarrhoea from emotions – **anticipation**, **apprehension**, **fear**; before a **panic attack**; from eating **sugar**

- Worse immediately after **drinking**; eating **cold food**; from lying on **right side**

- Better for burping; fresh, **cold air**

Arsenicum Album

- **Loose and watery** stools; severe **cramping** in abdomen; **burning** pain when defecating; nausea and **vomiting**; **restlessness**; weakness and **exhaustion**; **very chilly**; thirsty for **small sips** of water; **anxiety** and **despair**; craves **company**

- Food poisoning from **dirty water**, **ice cream**, **meat**, **shellfish**, **watery fruits** or **rotten vegetables**

- Worse for the **cold**; around **midnight**; with the thought or smell of **food**

- Better for **warm applications**; with **warm drinks**

Bryonia

- **Cramping**; sore abdomen; **gushing** diarrhoea; **yellow, mushy, foul-smelling** stools; **burning** anus after defecation; **irritable**; **thirsty** for large quantities of water; **dry** mouth and lips

- Diarrhoea from **hot weather**; from **cooling down too rapidly** after being very hot; from eating ice and ice cream when feeling very hot

- Worse in the **morning**; from **any slight movement**; after **cold drinks** in hot weather

- Better for **hard pressure**, e.g. holding the abdomen; lying on the painful area; being **quiet**; being **alone**; **staying still**

Gelsemium

- **Painless** defecation; **yellow** stools; feeling of **emptiness** in stomach; stomach cramps; **exhaustion** and **weakness**; **dullness** of mind; **trembling**

- Diarrhoea from **anticipation**, stage fright, bad news or shock

- Worse with strong **emotions**; in damp or humid weather

- Better for **bending forwards**; lying down quietly; **reclining** with head held high

Nux Vomica

- **Cramping**; painful defecation; frequent urge to defecate; gas and **bloating**; **griping** pains; **constant discomfort in rectum**; feeling **unfinished** after defecation, as if stool remains; **irritable**; **oversensitive**; **hypochondria**

- Diarrhoea from rich food or **alcohol**; antibiotics; overuse of **laxatives**; and colic in **babies** caused by breast-feeding mother's overstimulating diet

- Worse from **overindulgence**; strong odours; touch; **tight-fitting clothes**; in the **morning**

- Better for **heat**; warmth on the abdomen; **after passing stools** (for a short time)

Phosphorus

- **Very watery**, **painless** diarrhoea; **very smelly**, loose stools; flatulence; **exhaustion** and weakness; **burning** pains in the rectum; sensation of anus being open; **anxiety**

- Diarrhoea from a **fright** or from getting wet

- Worse from **getting wet** in hot weather; eating **warm food**

- Better for **company** and sympathy; **sleep**; **cold** food and drink

Podophyllum

- Stomach **cramping** and **gurgling**; **profuse**, **putrid**, **watery** stools; **green**, **yellow** stools containing **undigested food**; painless, **gushing** diarrhoea; explosive gas; constant nausea with foul-smelling burps; weakness; **thirst** for large quantities of water

- **Teething** children with hot glowing cheeks and loose stools, strong desire to **press their gums on hard things**

- Worse in the **early morning**, between 4 a.m. and 5 a.m.; after **eating and drinking**; during a hot summer

- Better for **applied heat** to the abdomen; lying down on the abdomen; from **rubbing** the liver region

Pulsatilla

- Heavy sensation of **stone in stomach**; sensitive digestion; **changeable symptoms**, stools are different every time; **watery** stools; **shy**, emotional, **tearful**; craves affection and company; **thirstless**; feel chilly

- Diarrhoea after eating **fats**, pork, **creamy food**, pastries, **ice cream** and eggs

- Worse during or after **menstruation**; from eating rich foods; strong emotions; at night (especially **twilight**)

- Better in **open air**; with **cold drinks** and food

Sulphur

- Loose and foul-smelling stools, like **rotten eggs**; painless defecation; **urgent**, early morning rush to toilet; **itching, redness, burning** of anus; feels **hot** and overheats easily

- Worse from **heat**; drinking **milk**; eating **sweet food**; in the **early morning**

- Better in **open air**

OTHER HOME REMEDIES

Ginger tea

Ginger has anti-inflammatory properties and can aid digestion. To soothe the stomach, boil slices of fresh ginger in water, strain and drink the tea.

Peppermint tea

Peppermint has antispasmodic properties that can help relieve the spasms of the digestive tract that accompany diarrhoea.

Ceylon cinnamon

Cinnamon is known for its anti-inflammatory properties, which may reduce inflammation in the digestive tract, alleviating the discomfort associated with diarrhoea. Additionally, cinnamon can help soothe and relax the muscles of the digestive tract, minimizing spasms that often accompany diarrhoea.

Prepare cinnamon tea by adding half a teaspoon of ground cinnamon to a cup of boiling water. Let the tea cool slightly before drinking and consider adding honey to enhance the flavour.

EARACHE

Earache is common in young children and is often linked to teething or a cold. Although it can be very painful, it's not usually a sign of a serious condition. Ear pain can occur in one or both ears. Ear infections are a frequent cause of earache in children and typically start to improve within a few days.

Signs of earache include:

- Irritability or restlessness
- Tugging at or rubbing the ear
- Not responding to certain sounds
- Fever, particularly with a temperature of 38°C (100.4°F)
- Loss of or no appetite
- Experiencing issues with balance

Actions that may help:

- Press a warm or cold wet flannel to the ear.
- Sit upright to relieve pressure in the ear.
- Chew on something to relieve the air pressure in the ear.

Seek help from a qualified practitioner:

- If the earache does not get better within three days
- If you have a very high temperature over 40°C (102°F)
- If there is pus or blood coming from the ear
- If there is swelling behind the ear
- If you have a severe earache that stops suddenly: this could be a perforated eardrum

HOMEOPATHIC REMEDIES

Aconite

- **Sudden onset** of pain in ear; **bright red**, swollen ear, **hot** to the touch; **tingling** and **buzzing** feeling; high fever; unbearable **sharp** pains; agitation; great **anxiety**; feeling of **drop of water in left ear**; restlessness; very **sensitive to noise**
- Use for earache triggered by **dry**, **cold winds**; from getting very cold; from **shock** or **fright**
- Worse at night (especially **midnight**); from being **chilled**; touch; noise
- Better for **being still**

Belladonna

- **Red** ear or cheek; **sudden onset with fever**; **throbbing**, pulsating pain; **humming** or **banging** sounds; hearing very acute on **right side**; **swollen glands** around ear and neck; **extreme pain, cries out** in sleep; ear feels **hot** inside and outside; **dilated** pupils; **glassy** eyes; cold hands and feet; craves **lemonade**

- Worse at **night**; in bed; from **heat**; jarring motion; at 3 p.m.

- Better for **wrapping up** warm; from **bending head backwards**

Chamomilla

- Sharp **stitch-like** pains; **soreness, swelling, heat; very sensitive to cold winds**; ear feels blocked; roaring noise like **rushing water**; sensation of hot water pouring out of ear; **one cheek pale, the other red**; frantic and **screaming** from **intolerable pain**; very **angry; despairing**; indecisive

- Whining, restless, **teething children** that can't be consoled

- Worse at night; from **touch** or being examined; from **cold air**

- Better from being **carried** or **rocked**; any **motion**; with **cold applications**

Hepar Sulph

- Leaking **yellow pus**, foul-smelling (like old cheese); **sensitive to touch; splinter-like pain**; deafness from accumulation of pus; roaring noises; **very chilly**; sensitive to cold of any kind; smelly breath; hypersensitive; **irritable**

- Use for **deeper infections** in ear canal; **middle ear** infections; earache triggered by exposure to cold or wind

- Worse from lying on painful side; **cold draughts**; at **night**

- Better with **warmth** to the ear; **covering** the ear

Merc Sol

- Shooting pains in **right ear**; pain extends from ear to teeth to throat; hot, red, swollen ear; **thick, yellow** discharge; sensation of **cold water running from ear**; sore throat; **metallic taste**; excessive saliva; smelly breath

- Use for more **advanced infections**, with pus

- Worse from **heat of the bed**; at night; from **swallowing**; lying on the **right side**

- Better for **cold applications**; **rest**

Pulsatilla

- **Thick, bland**, copious **yellow** discharge; **difficulty hearing**; ear feels **blocked up**; red, hot, swollen ear; thirstless; changeable symptoms; craves **affection** and sympathy; **tearful** and **clingy**

- Use for earache with or following **a cold**, congested with mucus

- Worse in the evening; at **night**; from being left alone; with heat; in **warm, stuffy rooms**

- Better for **cool air**

Silica

- **Left-sided**, perforated eardrum; **deafness**; **blocked up** feeling; foul-smelling, cheesy discharge; **crusts around ear**; itching of ears when swallowing; **hissing** or **roaring** noises; physical weakness and tiredness; **chilliness**

- Use for chronic ear infections; ear infection following vaccination (acute reaction often accompanied by a fever); **middle and later**

stages of a cold accompanied by ear infection; sickly, shy and timid children who get repeated ear infections

- Worse for cold air; **draughts**
- Better for **yawning; swallowing**

Silica is beneficial for treating chronic ear infections and for the middle and later stages of a cold if accompanied by an ear infection.

ABC (Aconite, Belladonna, Chamomilla) combination remedy 30c

This combination remedy is effective for sudden, intense earaches with no clear cause. It's particularly useful for urgent, middle-of-the-night scenarios as it can often deal with the earache pain straight away. After the pain has subsided, using one of the other remedies may be appropriate.

OTHER HOME REMEDIES

Olive oil

A few drops of lukewarm olive oil in the affected ear can help soothe earache. Olive oil can lubricate and help protect the ear from infections. Ensure the oil is warm to the touch but not hot.

Garlic

Garlic has natural antimicrobial properties and can act as a pain reliever. To make garlic oil, crush a garlic clove and mix it with a spoonful of warm (not hot) olive or sesame oil. Let it sit for a few minutes, then strain it. Apply a few drops of this mixture into the affected ear. Be sure the mixture is not too hot to avoid burning the ear canal.

FEVERS

A fever is a temporary rise in body temperature that on a thermometer reads 38°C (100.4°F) or higher. It's one of the initial responses from the immune system and usually happens at the start of an acute disease such as a cold, flu, childhood disease or microbial infection. A fever can result from various causes and is not always indicative of a serious condition.

Signs of fever include:

- Feeling hot
- Skin that feels hot to the touch, particularly on the forehead
- Tiredness
- Hot and cold chills in the neck and back
- Shivering
- Excessive sweating
- Flushed face

Actions that may help:

- Drink plenty of fluids to avoid dehydration.

- Wear comfortable clothing.

- Using tepid water, sponge down small areas of the body.

Seek medical advice for a persistent fever and an exceptionally high fever over 40°C (102°F).

HOMEOPATHIC REMEDIES

Aconite

- **First signs**; **sudden onset**; **dry, burning skin**; **high fever**; chills and shivering ; red, hot, flushed face; **one cheek red, the other pale**; very thirsty; contracted pupils; **restlessness; anxiety**

- Fevers from **dry, cold winds**; getting very cold; a **shock** or **fright**

- Worse in the evening; at **midnight**; from **touch**; motion; the cold

- Better from resting; in **open air**; being **uncovered** in bed

Arsenicum Album

- **Burning**, intermittent fever; **restlessness**; violent chill; teeth chattering; severe shivering; **exhaustion** and **weakness; anxiety; despair**; thirsty for **small sips**

- Worse around **midnight**; with **cold**; motion; in **open air**

- Better from **heat**; company

Belladonna

- **Sudden** high fever; **throbbing**, pulsating, **hears heartbeat** in ears; **bounding pulse**; hot, **dry** skin; **burning** heat without chills;

flushed, red face or very pale; **dilated, glassy pupils**; delirium and **hallucinations**; eyes very **sensitive to light**; **hot head, cold limbs**, ice cold feet; drowsy and limp; **thirstless**; craves **lemons**

- Worse in the **afternoon** (around 3 p.m.); from jarring motion; **noise**; light

- Better from light bed coverings; **bed rest**; being in a **dark room**

Bryonia

- **Slow onset** over a few days; heat alternates with chills; dry, **painful cough**; severe chills and violent **shivering**; sweaty; **muscular aches** and pains; splitting **frontal headaches**; **dry throat**, mouth, lips; **thirsty** for large quantities of water; **irritable**

- Worse in the **evening** (around 9 p.m.); with **any movement** (even of the eyes); in cold, wet weather; in autumn; when **eating**

- Better from **lying still**; drinking **cold water**; being **quiet**

Chamomilla

- **One cheek red, the other pale**; sweaty head; **diarrhoea** with **grass-green stools** like chopped eggs and spinach; irritable; **demanding**; hot and bothered; indecisive; impulsive; thirsty; **restlessness**

- Fever with **strong pain** in conditions such as **teething** or **earache** in **children**

- Worse from being **uncovered**; at **night** (between 9 p.m. and midnight); being **looked at**

- Better when **carried**; **rocked**; from **any motion**; **cold applications**

Ferrum Phos

- **Beginning stages**; **slow onset** over a few days; low-grade fever; depletion and exhaustion; **lethargic**; dry heat without chill; **sore throat**; **flushed, red** or **pale** skin; frequent sweats and shivering; thirsty for cold drinks; cold hands and feet; craves **sour** things

- Fevers with **lack of characteristic symptoms** or of **unknown** origin

- Worse between 4 a.m. and 6 a.m.; in **open air**; from **touch**

- Better with **cold applications**; **gentle motion**

Gelsemium

- **Slow onset**, flu-like fever; **aching** and **heaviness**; very **weak** and **trembling limbs**; chill in hands and feet; extreme **exhaustion**; **dizziness**; **drowsiness**; flushed face; dark red, dull skin; **droopy eyelids**; chills up and down the **back**; thirstless

- Worse from thinking about illness; with **motion**; talking

- Better after **urination**; rest; with **heat**

Pulsatilla

- **Dry heat**; no sweat; some parts of body feel hot, others feel cold; **symptoms constantly change**; chilliness but **aversion to heat**; one-sided coldness; burning hot at night; gastric upset; **thirstless**; craves affection and **sympathy**; tearful; **clingy**

- **Childhood** fevers that accompany childhood diseases and earaches

- Worse in the evening (around **twilight**); from being left **alone**; with **heat**, especially overheated, stuffy rooms

- Better in **open air**

OTHER HOME REMEDIES

Basil

This herb is remarkably effective in treating fevers. Boil a handful of basil leaves in water and drink the tea two or three times a day. For more flavour, add ginger and/or honey.

Garlic

Garlic is well known for its antibacterial and anti-inflammatory properties. These qualities make garlic a powerful tool in reducing fever, as well as clearing the bacteria that causes a fever.

Crush one clove of garlic and steep it in a cup of hot water for 10 minutes before straining. Drinking this garlic-infused water at least twice a day can be effective in treating a fever.

FOOD POISONING

Food poisoning happens when food is consumed that has been contaminated with bacteria or viruses due to improper handling, storage or preparation. Although it's usually not serious and tends to go away within a week, the elderly, young children and pregnant women are at higher risk of complications. Symptoms typically appear within 24 hours to three days after consuming contaminated food (but it can take longer) and most cases resolve within one to five days.

Food can be contaminated by:

- Improper cooking or inadequate reheating

- Incorrect storage, such as failure to freeze or refrigerate food correctly

- Handling by someone who is sick or hasn't washed their hands thoroughly

- Consumption past the food's expiration or 'use by' date

Signs of food poisoning include:

- Nausea and/or vomiting

- Diarrhoea

- Abdominal cramps

- Fever, specifically a temperature higher than 38°C (100.4°F)

- Overall malaise, including fatigue, body aches and chills

Actions that may help:

- Drink plenty of fluids. It's important to stay hydrated to prevent dehydration.

- Stay at home and rest.

- Follow the BRAT diet – bananas, rice, applesauce and toast.

- Try an electrolyte replacement solution.

When to seek medical help:

- Fever over 40°C (102°F)

- Diarrhoea that is bloody and lasts over three days

- Frequent vomiting, unable to keep liquids down

- Dehydration with little or no urination

HOMEOPATHIC REMEDIES

Arsenicum Album

- Frequent diarrhoea; loose, watery, offensive-smelling stools; nausea; vomiting; severe cramping pain in abdomen; **burning pain on defecating**; **weakness** and **exhaustion**; **very chilly**; **restlessness**; **anxiety** and **despair**; craves **company**

- Food poisoning from **bad meat**; shellfish; watery fruits or vegetables; contaminated water; eating something very cold (like ice cream) on a hot day

- Worse around **midnight** (between 11 p.m. and 2 a.m.); from cold; from thought or smell of food

- Better for warm applications; **small sips of warm drinks**

If Arsenicum Album hasn't helped, try using China instead, especially if bloating is a symptom.

Carbo Veg

- Severe, foul-smelling diarrhoea (cadaver odour); extreme **weakness**, state of **collapse**; **listless** and **indifferent**; **bloated** stomach; belching; extreme flatulence; trapped wind; **cramping** in abdomen; hands and feet feel **icy cold**; breathless

- Food poisoning from fish, ice water, vegetables

- Worse from **hot, stuffy rooms**; being covered; lying down; eating **fatty foods**

- Better for **belching**; sitting up; in **open air**; with cold drinks

China

- Profuse, painless 'traveller's' diarrhoea; vomiting; **dehydration**; **weakness**; **bloated, distended with gas**; regurgitation of food; **indigestion** leaves **sour taste**; **stomach feels cold** and full after small amount of food; food and water **tastes bitter**; **irritable**; oversensitive to noise; very chilly

- Food poisoning from fish, meat, milk, impure water, fruit (fermentation in stomach)
- Worse from **slight touch**; **cold**; at night; after meals; with **loss of fluids**
- Better for warmth; **hard pressure**, e.g. massage; in open air; with **loose clothes**

Ipecac

- **Persistent nausea** and **vomiting**; loathing of **sight or smell of food**; **profuse saliva**; hot head and cold legs; diarrhoea with offensive-smelling, **frothy, black, sticky stools**; severe cramps; colic
- Worse from **lying down**; with warmth; **ice cream**; **pork**; **cold drinks**
- Better for rest; **closing eyes**; being in **open air**

Nux Vomica

- Cramping; frequent, painful diarrhoea, unfinished feeling; **griping pains**; **constant uneasiness**; gas; distension; feels **chilly**; **irritable**; **oversensitive**; **hypochondria**
- Worse from **noise**; smells; touch; cold; overindulgence (**rich food** or **alcohol**); antibiotics; overuse of **laxatives**; **tight-fitting clothes**; in the morning
- Better for **heat** and warmth on abdomen; **after passing stools** (for a short time)

Pulsatilla

- Watery diarrhoea; **heavy sensation** in stomach; **thirstless**; sensitive digestive tract; changeable symptoms, **stools vary** in type; timid, **emotional**, tearful; craves affection and company

- Food poisoning from rich food, **fatty food, pork, creamy food,** pastries, **ice cream, eggs**

- Worse in **hot, stuffy rooms**; with strong emotions; at night (around **twilight**)

- Better in **open air**; with **cold drinks** and food

OTHER HOME REMEDIES

Ginger tea

Ginger is rich in compounds that can help to alleviate nausea and vomiting. As an anti-inflammatory, it can soothe stomach cramps and ease flatulence. Studies have also shown that ginger is effective at stopping diarrhoea. To make ginger tea, boil slices of fresh ginger in water, strain and then drink the tea.

Peppermint

Peppermint tea can relax the intestinal muscles, reducing the pain from the stomach cramps that often accompany diarrhoea. Smelling peppermint oil can help relieve nausea and vomiting.

Fennel tea

Fennel has properties that can promote good digestion, reduce the tendency of vomiting and help alleviate nausea. Consuming fennel seeds in the form of tea can be beneficial. Research has shown that fennel can inhibit the growth of certain bacteria, making it useful in treating food poisoning. Additionally, it may help reduce gas, bloating and stomach cramps.

Ceylon cinnamon

Cinnamon is known for its anti-inflammatory and antimicrobial qualities which may alleviate the discomfort associated with diarrhoea. Cinnamon can help relax the digestive tract muscles, soothing the spasms that accompany diarrhoea. Add half a teaspoon of ground cinnamon to a cup of hot water and add honey to sweeten if necessary.

GRIEF AND LOSS

Grief is the profound emotional response to loss, particularly to the loss of someone or something to which a bond was formed. It invokes shock, anger, guilt, despair and loneliness. Grief is a natural process that differs greatly from person to person in its duration and expression.

Signs of acute grief include:

- Shock and disbelief

- Tearfulness

- Sadness and sorrow

- Fear and anguish

- Longing

- Insomnia

- Loss of appetite

Actions that may help:

- Express feelings and emotions and avoid suppressing them.

- Write about thoughts and feelings in a journal.

- Talk to friends, family, a therapist or join a support group.

- Maintain a consistent daily routine.

- Eat well and exercise.

If grief becomes overwhelming and too much to bear, seek advice from a healthcare professional who is experienced in grief counselling.

HOMEOPATHIC REMEDIES

Ignatia

- Distressed; **tearful**; unhappy; highly emotional; outbursts of **sobbing**; **controlled**, tries to keep emotion in; frequent **deep sighing**; oversensitive; **mood swings**; sensation of **lump in throat**; insomnia

- **Grief** after losing a person or object that was very dear; from **disappointment**

- Worse with **consolation**; **coffee**; tobacco smoke; stimulants

- Better with **swallowing**; being **alone**

Natrum Mur

- **Closed, shutdown, stoic**; keeps busy; **cannot cry** in front of others; craves **salt**

- **Long-standing** grief; or grief from **loss, deep disappointment**, rejection

- Worse from **consolation**; strong emotions; exposure to salty sea air

- Better in **open air**; from fasting; deep breathing; **tight-fitting clothing**

Phos-ac

- **Apathy; exhaustion; weakness**; lack of emotion; talks in a **monotone voice**; overwhelmed; traumatized; dullness of mind and dazed; aversion to loved ones; **indifferent** to life; desires **solitude**; crushing, heavy pain on top of head; loss of appetite but **craves fizzy drinks** and juicy, refreshing foods

- Use for **homesickness**

- Worse from being talked to; **cold draughts**

- Better for **short naps**; from warmth

Pulsatilla

- **Changeable moods**; highly **sensitive**; **weeps easily** whether from joy or sadness; feels f**orsaken**; fears being **unloved**; craves **affection**, attention, sympathy and **company**; thirstless

- Grief from **abandonment**

- Worse for warm, **stuffy rooms**

- Better for being **consoled**, held or hugged; in cool, fresh, **open air**

OTHER HOME REMEDIES

Rescue Remedy

Rescue Remedy is a blend of five of the original 38 Bach flower remedies that can help with feelings of panic, distress and loss. Put four drops of Rescue Remedy directly on the tongue or add four drops to water and sip at intervals. Repeat as necessary.

Chamomile tea

Chamomile contains compounds with sedative effects. These effects restore the ability to rest and sleep, which is essential during times of intense emotional distress. Chamomile's calming and soothing effects can also help manage grief, stress and anxiety.

HAY FEVER

Hay fever is an allergic reaction to grass or pollen. It can affect people at different times of the year depending on degree of sensitivity. Sufferers can be reactive to tree pollen in the spring, grass pollen in late spring and early summer or pollen from weeds in autumn. It affects many people and symptoms can vary from year to year.

Signs of hay fever include:

- Itchy, red and watery eyes

- Streaming or stuffed up nose

- Sneezing fits

- Itchy nose and throat

Actions that may help:

- Keep the windows and doors closed to minimize pollen exposure, especially on windy days or when the pollen count is high.

- Wear wraparound sunglasses when outside to protect the eyes from pollen.

- When returning from outside, remove clothes and shower to rinse the pollen from hair and skin.

- Nasal irrigation is a quick, inexpensive and effective way to ease symptoms. Rinse nasal passages with saline solution to relieve congestion and flush out mucus and allergens from your nose.

Chronic hay fever sufferers should seek treatment from a qualified practitioner to deal with the underlying cause.

HOMEOPATHIC REMEDIES

Allium Cepa

- **Watery**, bland nasal discharge (no taste or colour) or **burning** discharge; **sneezing**; nose feels **raw**; head feels dull and **bunged up**; itching in nose, back of throat and roof of mouth; red eyes, **sensitive to light**; profuse watery, burning tears; sensitive to **peach skin** and odour of flowers
- Hay fever that predominantly affects the **nose**
- Worse in **warm rooms**
- Better in cool, **open air**

Arsenicum Album

- **Burning** in eyes and nose; nose constantly running with **acrid**, watery discharge; **sore, chapped**, itching, flaking skin around nose; sneezing; **asthma**, coughing, wheezing; shortness of breath
- Worse when outdoors; in **mid-summer**; lying down; with cold air; at **midnight**
- Better when **sitting up**; **indoors**

Arundo

- **Burning** and annoying **itching** of eyes, **roof of mouth, nostrils**; pain at **bridge** of nose; loss of smell; sneezing; **clear mucus**, can become **green** and **thick**; constant **thirst**, especially on waking; **water tastes bad**

Euphrasia

- Eyes constantly water; **acrid** and **burning tears**; sensation of **sand in eyes**; bland nasal discharge; nose **drips** during the day but **blocked up** at night; **splitting pain** and pressure across forehead

- Hay fever that predominantly affects the **eyes**

- Worse with **sunlight**; wind

- Better in open air; with **wiping** eyes; **blinking**

Natrum Mur

- Violent **sneezing**; runny nose; thin nasal discharge, like **egg white**; **itching, burning**, watering eyes; **photophobia**; craves **salt**

- Worse with **sunlight**

- Better with **open air**; washing face in **cold water**

Nux Vomica

- **Sneezing**; **runny nose** in the day and **stuffed up** at night; blocked nose on **one side**; wheezing; clothes feel too tight; **irritable**; impatient

- Worse at **night**; outdoors; from **fullness in stomach**

- Better for **blowing nose** to clear discharge

Pulsatilla

- **Thick**, **bland** nasal discharge; stuffed up nose; **itching**, **burning**, watering eyes; **inflamed** eyelids; eyelashes stuck with thick, **yellow** mucus; loss of taste and/or smell

- Worse in **hot**, stuffy rooms

- Better **outside**; in open air

Sabadilla

- **Spasmodic** bouts of loud sneezing; runny nose; copious, watery nasal discharge; itching and **tingling** in nose and **roof of mouth**; redness and burning in eyes, lots of tears; **dry** mouth but **thirstless**; severe sinus pain over the eyes; blocked nose, changes side; sensitive to smell; **nasal inflammation**

- Worse from **cold air**; odours of **flowers**; newly **cut grass**; smell of **garlic**

- Better in a **warm room**; being **wrapped up**; being **indoors**; in open air

Wyethia

- **Itching** of **nose, throat** and **roof of mouth**; sneezing; runny nose; dry, swollen throat; **difficulty swallowing**; constant desire to **clear the throat** or swallow; **pricking** or dry sensation in sinuses; sensation of **something in nasal passages**; **irritable, dry cough**

- Hay fever that goes to the **lungs**

- Worse in **afternoon**; with **exercise**

- Nothing seems to ease the symptoms

Mixed Pollen

Mixed Pollen is a combination remedy that contains a mixture of grasses, cereals, early and mid-blossom trees and weeds. This can be taken to lessen sensitivity to hay fever symptoms and/or along with other remedies for specific symptoms associated with hay fever.

OTHER HOME REMEDIES

Local honey

Many people believe that eating local honey helps them with their hay fever as it encourages their body to adapt to the local pollen in the area where they live.

Chamomile tea

Chamomile is well known for its antihistamine properties. Chamomile tea can also be used as an eye compress if the eyes are inflamed. This method is especially helpful for soothing swollen, red eyes, providing a cooling and calming effect.

Brew the tea, let it cool down and soak a clean cloth or cotton wool pad in the tea. Alternatively use the moist tea bags as a compress.

HEADACHES

Headaches are a common condition marked by pain or discomfort in the head, scalp or neck. There are lots of different types of headaches, including tension headaches, migraines, cluster headaches and sinus headaches. Each type has its own triggers and characteristics – it's important to understand the underlying cause to choose the most effective homeopathic remedy for relief.

Signs of a headache include:

- Pain in the head or face (localized or widespread)

- Sensitivity to light (photophobia) or sound

- Pressure or tightness in the head

- Nausea or vomiting

- Blurred vision, visual disturbances or auras

- Stiff neck or muscle tension

- Fatigue or lethargy

- Irritability or mood changes

- Dizziness or light-headedness

- Nasal congestion or runny nose

- Difficulty concentrating

- Scalp tenderness

Some common causes of headaches include:

- Having a cold or flu

- Stress or strong emotions

- Drinking too much alcohol

- Bad posture

- Eyesight problems or eye strain

- Not eating regular meals

- Not drinking enough fluids (dehydration)

- Too much sun/sunstroke

- Menstruation or menopause

- Side effects from conventional medications

Actions that may help:

- Drink plenty of water to stay hydrated.

- Rest in a quiet, dark room to reduce sensory stimulation.

- Apply a cold or warm compress.

- Practise relaxation techniques, such as deep breathing, meditation or yoga.

Headaches are common and not usually a sign of something serious. However, you should seek urgent medical attention if:

- You have a head injury, e.g. from a fall or accident

- The headache comes on suddenly and is extremely painful

- You experience problems speaking or remembering things

- You feel drowsy or confused

- You experience loss of vision

- You have a very high temperature and symptoms of meningitis

HOMEOPATHIC REMEDIES

Belladonna

- **Congestive** headaches with red face and rush of blood to head; **sudden onset**; **throbbing**, hammering pain in temples, **right-sided**; pain, fullness, throbbing and heat in forehead; sensitive to **draughts**, cold air, **cutting or washing hair**; usually starts **late afternoon** and continues into night

- Headaches from too much sun or **sunstroke**

- Worse for **motion**, especially **jarring**; **noise**; light

- Better for **pressure**; bending head backwards; laying hand on head

Bryonia

- Bursting, splitting frontal headaches; **pressure** in head, as if too full; pain over **left eye** going to back of head; scalp very sensitive to touch; **very thirsty** with dry lips; **irritable**; doesn't want to talk

- Worse from **any movement**, even **moving eyes**; from stooping

- Better with firm pressure; from **lying still** in a dark room; cold applications; being alone

Cocculus

- **Pain in back of head** or nape of neck; nausea and vomiting; **strange sensations**, such as hollow feeling in head or opening and shutting sensation at back of head; feeling as if **skull will burst**; **very tired** from mental or physical strain; unable to bear the slightest light or noise

- Headaches accompanying **motion sickness**; after **travelling**, especially long journeys; from lack of sleep, e.g. from over-studying or night nursing

- Worse from lying down; **lack of sleep**; motion; coffee; cold air; touch; **pressure**

- Better from **bending backwards**; sitting; being quiet; in a warm room

Gelsemium

- Sensation of a **band around head** or pain at back of head; right-sided pain; pain in temple extending into ear; dull, heavy ache with **heavy eyelids**; blurred vision; **mental dullness** with poor concentration; faintness and trembling; fatigue; **drowsiness**; **apathy**; wants to be quiet and left alone; **thirstless**

- Headaches from being **nervous** or **excited**; from **anticipation** or hearing **bad news**; from onset of **influenza**

- Worse from mental exertion; heat of sun; lying with **head low**

- Better with pressure; **urination**; from **head raised high** on pillow

Ignatia

- Pain in small, **targeted area**; sensation of nail being driven out through side of head; throbbing pains in forehead and over eyes; oversensitive to pain; very **emotional**; frequent **sighing**

- Headaches from emotional **shock, grief** or **disappointment**

- Worse with **strong emotions**; from **tobacco smoke**; **coffee**; alcohol; open air; stooping

- Better when **eating**; from being quiet; being left alone; with pressure

Natrum Mur

- Bursting, **blinding** pain; sensation of a thousand little hammers knocking on brain; pain over eyes and top of head; **visual disturbances** and **sensitivity to light**

- Headaches from **strong emotions**, such as **grief** or **disappointed love**; from the heat of the sun

- Worse on waking; with **sunlight**; from **sunrise to sunset**

- Better with **sleep**; pressure; from lying with head high; sitting still

Nux Vomica

- Pain in back of head or over eyes with **vertigo**; frontal headache with desire to press head against something; brain feels **bruised**; pressing pain on top of head, sensation of nail being driven in; very chilly; **hypersensitive**; **irritated by everything**

- Headaches from **toxicity**; drugs or alcohol **hangover**

- Worse with cold draughts; disturbed sleep; noise; light; touch; **rich food**; **alcohol**; constipation

- Better for **warmth**; rest; hot drinks

Pulsatilla

- **One-sided** headache; pain in right temple; throbbing, congestive headache; heat in head; pressure on top of head, **heavy sensation**; difficult holding head upright; oversensitive to pain; **thirstless**; emotional; **tearful**

- Headaches from **puberty** in females; from **menstruation**, usually before flow begins; from overeating **fatty foods**, such as pastries and ice cream

- Worse at **twilight**; from **rich food**; in **warm**, **stuffy rooms**

- Better for walking in **open air**; rubbing; pressure

Sanguinaria

- **Periodical** headaches that return nightly or weekly; pain at **back of head** like a 'flash of lightning', **extending to right eye**; sensation as if eyes might pop out; nausea, relieved by vomiting; **flushes of heat to the face** with **redness of cheeks**

- Headaches from the sun; from **going without food**; from **menopause**

- Worse on **right side**; from **motion**; during the day until the evening; at 3 a.m.

- Better with **sleep**; **darkness**; cool air

OTHER HOME REMEDIES

Peppermint oil

Peppermint oil is one of the most widely used essential oils for headaches. It contains menthol, which has a cooling effect that can help relax muscles and reduce pain. It's particularly effective for tension headaches.

Mix a few drops of peppermint oil with a carrier oil (like coconut, almond, olive or jojoba oil) and apply it to the temples, forehead or back of the neck. You can also inhale the aroma directly from the bottle or use it in a diffuser.

Lavender oil

Lavender oil is known for its calming and relaxing properties, making it useful for stress-related headaches and migraines. It can help ease tension and promote better sleep, which can also help to prevent headaches.

Inhale lavender oil directly or diffuse it into your room. You can also dilute it with a carrier oil and apply it to your temples or wrists.

Ginger tea

Ginger is known for its anti-inflammatory and pain-relieving properties, making it useful for reducing pain from headaches, especially migraines. It's also effective in alleviating nausea, a common symptom associated with migraines.

Add fresh ginger slices to boiling water and let the tea steep for about 10 minutes before drinking. You can also use ginger tea bags for a quicker option.

Coriander seeds

Coriander seeds have been used in traditional medicine to relieve sinus headaches. The seeds help reduce inflammation and clear nasal congestion, which can alleviate sinus pressure.

Steep coriander seeds in hot water. Then you can either drink the tea or inhale the steam to clear your sinuses.

HEAD LICE (NITS)

Head lice are parasitic insects that live in the hair. Nits are the white, empty eggshells left attached to the hair once the lice have hatched. Female lice can live up to 40 days, in which time they can lay hundreds of eggs. Head lice are transferred from head-to-head contact and are especially common in young children as they play near one another. To determine if you have head lice, apply conditioner to the hair and comb through using a nit comb.

Signs of head lice include:

- Very itchy scalp
- Crawling sensation of the scalp
- Visible lice crawling in the hair
- Finding eggs that look like white specs or dandruff in the hair
- Irritability
- Soreness and redness of the scalp from persistent itching

Actions that may help:

- The best way to get rid of head lice is to remove them manually from the hair for 10–14 days to prevent reinfestation.

- To remove the lice and nits, apply hair conditioner or coconut oil to the hair and use a fine-tooth comb (nit comb) to comb through the hair thoroughly. The lice are mostly found in the hairline at the back of the neck and around the ears, so comb these areas thoroughly. Repeat this process daily or on alternate days for 10 days to ensure you have removed both mature and newly hatched lice.

- Wash all bedding, clothing and other personal items that may have come into contact with the infested person's head. Dry these items on a high heat, e.g. in the tumble drier, to help kill any lice or eggs that may be present.

- Small children don't feel itchy until they are completely infested. To minimize spreading throughout the household, check other family members for lice and encourage them to avoid head-to-head contact with the infested person until the infestation is resolved.

HOMEOPATHIC REMEDY

Staphysagria 30c

- Use twice a week for head lice.

OTHER HOME REMEDIES

Tea tree oil and star anise oil

Mix a few drops of tea tree oil and star anise oil into a carrier oil (such as almond, coconut or olive oil) and massage the mixture into the scalp. Leave it for a few hours or overnight, and then comb through the hair with a fine-toothed metal comb to remove the lice and nits. Wipe the comb on a white cloth or kitchen towel to see the lice and nits that have been removed.

When finished, shampoo twice to remove the oil and then rinse with an apple cider vinegar dilution. Mix equal parts of apple cider vinegar and water in a spray bottle. Leave on the scalp for 5–10 minutes and then rinse with warm water.

Citronella oil

To prevent infestation, add a few drops of citronella oil to water in a spray bottle and spray onto the hair daily.

HOT FLUSHES (FLASHES)

———— ❧ ————

Many women encounter hot flushes during menopause, which may begin in the perimenopausal phase and persist for years after menstruation ceases. These flushes can occur unexpectedly, affecting the entire body, often accompanied by facial redness and sweating. They can happen at any time, day or night, and vary in intensity from mild and sporadic to severe and very frequent. It's believed that fluctuations in hormone levels disrupt the body's ability to regulate temperature, leading to these symptoms.

Signs of hot flushes include:

- Sudden sensation of warmth or heat in the body
- Flushed skin particularly on the face, neck and chest
- Blotchy rashes or patchy redness
- Nausea and dizziness
- Sweating
- Rapid heartbeat
- Anxiety and agitation
- Disturbed sleep

Actions that may help:

- Keep your environment cool.

- Wear lightweight, breathable clothing, such as cotton.

- Dress in layers so clothes can be removed if a hot flush comes on.

- Stay hydrated by drinking plenty of fluids.

- Limit food and drinks that can trigger a hot flush, such as spices, caffeine, hot drinks and alcohol.

- Exercise.

HOMEOPATHIC REMEDIES

Amylenum Nit

- Flushing, hot, **red face**; throbbing **pulsations** all over body; hot, **drenching sweats**; cold, clammy skin; lower part of body feels icy cold; **left-sided headaches**; throbbing and bursting sensation in head and ears; **violent heartbeat**; feeling of **pulsating veins**; constant desire to stretch the body; **anxiety**

- Worse with **heat**; in a stuffy, warm room; from **strong emotions**

- Better with **cold water**; open air; **exercise**

Belladonna

- **Sudden** hot flushes, come and go quickly; flushed face; dilated pupils; **right-sided headaches**; dry skin, **radiates heat**; **throbbing** and burning sensations; body sweats, head remains dry; **craves lemons** and lemonade

- Worse with **heat**; around **3 p.m.**
- Better for **light clothing**

Cimicifuga

- Hot flushes at **night** or **morning**; **depressed**, as if followed by a **black cloud**; aching; shooting soreness and pain in joints, muscles, nerves; **stiffness** and contraction in neck and back; **arthritis** affecting **large joints**; general bruised feeling all over; very chilly
- Worse with **touch**; wine; cold draughts; at night; with a **change in weather**
- Better in **open air**; with a **warm wrap**

Glonoinum

- Hot flushes **ascending from pit of stomach to top of head**; **pulsating** heat; **severe palpitations**; alternating between pale and flushed face; **perspiration on forehead and chest**; bursting, **pounding headache**, comes in waves; **heavy head**; **throbbing in temples**; intolerant of loved ones; dwells on past events and grievances
- Worse with **heat**; from laying head down; **movement**; walking; hot weather
- Better from **elevating head**; **cold applications**

Lachesis

- Rush of blood to the head; **flushes of heat**, **ascending** sensation; **cold feet**; feeling of **lump in throat** or **constriction**; throbbing, **burning head**, sensation of **weight**, pressure; bursting or pulsating headaches; **palpitations**; **jealous** and **suspicious**; emotional outbursts; reclusive and anti-social

- Worse on waking; from heat; **tight-fitting clothing**; anything **constricting**; alcohol; sun; lying on **left side**

- Better for **cold drinks**; in **open air**; with **pressure** on head

Sepia

- Rising heat through the body; **lack of warmth** in the body, chilly in a warm room; **anxiety**; profuse sweating; sudden **muscle weakness**; awakes at night with hot flushes; **very irritable**; sensitive; **worn out**; desire to be alone; **intolerant of loved ones**; **loss of libido**

- Worse from **cold air**; standing; **at night**

- Better when **warm**; busy; with **open air**; **exercise**

Sul-ac

- General **aggravation**; irritable, **angry**, **impatient**; severe hot flushes with perspiration and **trembling** all over; drenching sweats with **sour odour**; **weakness**; craves alcohol; very chilly, sensation of heat when eating **warm food**

- Worse towards the **evening**; during **sleep**; in **open air**

- Better in a **moderate temperature**; having **hot drinks**; being on the **coast**

Sulphur

- Sudden, violent, ascending, **throbbing** waves of heat throughout the whole body; profuse sweat at night with **smelly sulphur 'eggy' odour** under arms, hands and feet; **soles of feet burn** at night; **offensive-smelling perspiration on nape of neck** or back of head; wakes frequently, can't sleep between 2 a.m. and 5 a.m.

- Worse with heat; **warmth of bed**; humidity; after a bath; at night; **standing**

- Better with **open air**; lying on **right side**; sweating

OTHER HOME REMEDIES

Sage tea

Drinking a cup of sage tea can provide relief from the intensity and frequency of hot flushes as it may to help to balance fluctuating oestrogen levels.

Mint water

Add a few sprigs of fresh mint to cold water or drink cooled mint tea throughout the day to minimize the intensity of hot flushes.

Phytoestrogens

Foods rich in phytoestrogens, such as linseed (also known as flaxseed), can help minimize fluctuating oestrogen levels during menopause. Linseed must be ground up to maximize absorption and can be added to breakfast cereal, porridge, smoothies or yoghurt.

IMPETIGO

Impetigo is a highly contagious bacterial skin infection that is most common in young children. It can spread through direct contact with the sores, or by touching and sharing items, making it easy for children who play together to infect each other. The sores usually appear on the face, around the mouth and nose, but they can also spread to other parts of the body.

Impetigo remains contagious until the sores have crusted over and dried out. Treatment typically helps resolve impetigo within seven to 10 days. Although it's more common in young children, anyone can contract it.

Signs of impetigo include:

- Red sores or blisters around mouth or nose

- Pus-filled sores or blisters that can burst, leading to crusty, golden-brown patches

- Sores or blisters that are itchy and painful

Actions that may help:

- Avoid scratching the sores or blisters.

- Keep the affected area clean and dry.

- Wash hands frequently to stop the spread of infection.

- Apply a warm damp cloth to the affected area to ease discomfort.

HOMEOPATHIC REMEDIES

Ant Crud

- **Yellow, crusted** eruptions around **mouth**, nose and chin that burn and itch; **thick, hard, honey-coloured** scabs; **cracks in corners of mouth**; sore, dry, crusty nostrils; **white, thick coating** on tongue; very **irritable**, dislikes being **touched** or **looked at**; **gastric issues**, e.g. bloating after eating, constant belching

- Worse at **night**; with **heat from sunlight or bed coverings**; **cold bathing**

- Better in open air; with **moist, warm compresses**

Graphites

- Moist, crusty eruptions oozing with a **honey-like, sticky discharge**, pus or watery blood; eruptions begin **pale** in colour with itching, followed by scab formation and itching subsides; eruptions **slow to heal**; cracked, sore lips, mouth and nostrils

- Impetigo found in the **folds of the skin**: behind ears, neck, nose, corners of the mouth, mostly on the **left side**

- Worse with **heat**; at **night**

- Better in **open air**

Mezereum

- **Unbearable itching**; thick scabs **around the mouth**, crusting like chalk; oozing yellow, **thick pus under the scabs**; acrid, glue-like nasal discharge; eruptions **bleed on touch**; very sensitive to **cold**, even in warm room; overwhelming **anxiety**, felt in stomach

- Itching eruptions after **vaccination**

- Worse at **night** (evening to midnight); with **touch**; and from warmth of bed

- Better in open air; from **radiated heat source**

Rhus Tox

- **Dry, hot**, burning rash, small red spots, especially on **right side** of the body; red, **swollen**, itching skin that stings, like being pierced with **hot needles**; small crops of blisters in clusters around corners of mouth and chin; small, itchy blisters sore to the touch, ooze **foul-smelling, yellow pus**, thick crusts form over eruptions; swollen glands; sore throat; **restlessness** and anxiety in evening

- Worse if cold, wet or damp; at **midnight**; with **cold air**

- Better from applying **heat**; with hot compresses

Viola Tricolor

- Groups of pustules followed by scabs; thick scabs on **face** that crack and ooze yellow, watery pus; pus **hardens** like a **thick** gum; **burning** and **intolerable itching**, especially at night; cracked or sticky, **gummy crusts on scalp** that ooze yellow pus, **matting hair** together; urine can smell like **cat's pee**; frequent urge to urinate; high volume of urine

- Impetigo on face, head, chin, upper lip

- Worse in **winter**; with cold air; at night

- Nothing seems to ease the symptoms

OTHER HOME REMEDIES

Calendula

Calendula is a great addition to your first aid box, whether in the form of a herbal tincture or cream. Add a few drops of the herbal tincture to a small amount of cooled boiled water and bathe the affected area to promote healing, reduce inflammation and clear infection. Apply Calendula cream twice daily if the skin is cracked and sore.

Manuka honey

Many studies have shown that Manuka honey has antimicrobial properties, which may help kill the bacteria that cause impetigo. Apply the honey to the impetigo lesions, leave it on for 20 minutes and then wash it off with warm water.

INDIGESTION

Indigestion is discomfort or pain in the upper abdomen or chest after drinking or eating. Most people experience indigestion at some point in their lives, particularly those who smoke or are overweight. Other causes can include eating too quickly, consuming a large meal, eating fried or spicy foods or foods high in fat. Drinking excess amounts of coffee, tea or alcohol can also worsen indigestion. Additionally, mental or emotional stress can trigger indigestion.

Signs of indigestion include:

- Heartburn after eating or drinking

- Bloating and burping

- Nausea

- Feeling of pressure or fullness

- Bitter taste in the mouth

Actions that may help:

- Eat small meals, slowly.

- Avoid or cut down on eating rich, spicy and fried foods.

- Consume less tea, coffee and alcohol.

- Use a pillow to prop yourself up in bed at night.

- Reduce stress.

Chest pain could indicate a heart attack. Seek immediate medical attention if you are experiencing severe chest pain or pressure, arm or jaw pain or difficulty swallowing.

HOMEOPATHIC REMEDIES

Arsenicum Album

- **Burning pains** in stomach; vomiting; diarrhoea; heartburn with acid rising, burning throat; belching; hiccups; feeling **chilly**; **anxiety**; despair; **restlessness**

- Indigestion from consuming **vinegar**, **acids**, **ice cream** or **ice water**

- Worse from eating **cold foods**; drinking ice water; at night (between **11 p.m. and 2 a.m.**)

- Better from drinking **small sips of warm drinks** such as milk; eating little and often

Carbo Veg

- **Bloating** and **gas** with rancid, sour burps that give **temporary relief**; slow digestion, left with a **feeling of fullness or heaviness**; flatulence; abdominal **distension**

- Indigestion from **overindulging** in rich food and wine, especially in older individuals

- Worse for rich, fatty food; wine; butter; coffee; milk; **tight-fitting clothes** around the waist

- Better for belching; **open air**; **elevating feet**

Lycopodium

- Weak digestion; **excess gas**; **bloating**, particularly in lower abdomen **immediately after eating**; stomach **feels full** even after small amount of food; frequent, painful belching; sour burps

- Worse from tight-fitting clothes; between 4 p.m. and 8 p.m.; drinking **cold drinks**; eating bread

- Better from **belching**; motion; after midnight; with **warm food** and drinks

Nux Vomica

- Heartburn; bloating; **irritability**; **impatience**; anger; **sensitivity** to external environment

- Indigestion from **overeating**; alcohol; caffeine

- Worse in morning; when cold and uncovered; from noise, **alcohol**; tight-fitting clothes

- Better with heat; **hot drinks**, having a nap; lying down

Pulsatilla

- **Belching**; can **taste food** for a long time after eating; nausea; sensation of **stomach heaviness**; stomach feels **tight**, **must loosen clothing**; changeable mood; **craves open air**

- Indigestion after eating, especially rich, **fatty foods**

- Worse from eating **rich** foods; ice cream
- Better from drinking **cold drinks**; sitting or standing up; being outside

OTHER HOME REMEDIES

Fennel seeds

Fennel is well known for easing the symptoms of indigestion as it stimulates the secretion of digestive juices and enzymes. Make fennel tea by boiling half a teaspoon of fennel seeds in water for 5–10 minutes. Alternatively, chew a handful of dried fennel seeds after a meal, especially after eating foods that normally cause digestive discomfort.

Ginger

Ginger is a traditional remedy for digestive issues, including indigestion. Its natural anti-inflammatory and gastrointestinal soothing properties can help relieve symptoms like nausea and bloating. To soothe the stomach, boil slices of fresh ginger in water, strain and drink the tea.

INFLUENZA (FLU)

Influenza or flu can vary in severity. A person may feel unwell for a few days and recover quickly, but if they are run-down, chronically stressed or have low immunity, flu can be more serious and harder to resolve.

Signs of influenza can include:

- Rapid onset of fever and chills
- Sore throat
- Runny or stuffy nose
- Headache
- Loss of appetite
- Cough
- Aches and pains all over the body
- Fatigue
- Digestive upset including nausea, vomiting and diarrhoea

Actions that may help:

- Rest and sleep.

- Drink plenty of fluids, especially warm drinks and broth.

- Avoid sugary drinks and alcohol.

If there is no improvement after seven days, contact a qualified healthcare practitioner.

HOMEOPATHIC REMEDIES

Aconite

- **First signs** of influenza; **sudden onset**; dry, burning skin; high fever with a chill and shivering (fever and chill can alternate); red, hot, flushed face with one cheek red, the other pale; **restlessness**; contracted pupils; very thirsty when feverish or chilled; **anxiety**

- Influenza from **dry, cold winds**; getting very cold from **shock** or **fright**

- Worse in evening; around **midnight**; with touch; motion; cold

- Better with resting; in **open air**

Arsenicum Album

- Intermittent, **burning fever**, feels as if **hot water** runs through veins; internal **chills** with external heat and red cheeks, or internal heat with externally cold hands and feet; **vomiting**; **diarrhoea**; **extremely cold**, feels like **blood is ice**; exhaustion and **great weakness** from slightest exertion; dry cough, wheezing, breathlessness; **burning pain in chest**; **anxiety around health**; despair; urgent thirst, drinks in **sips, little and often**

- Influenza with gastroenteritis

- Worse in wet weather; with **cold, damp air**; around **midnight** (between 11 p.m. and 2 a.m.)

- Better with **heat**; company; open air; from sweating

Bryonia

- **Slow onset** over a few days; aches and pains in every muscle and joint; uncomfortable, **penetrating coldness** predominates; dry, **painful, hacking cough, holds the chest** to keep it still and stop pain; splitting **frontal headaches**; pain over left eye radiating to back of head; **dry throat**, mouth and lips; **thirsty** for large volume of water; very **irritable; despair**

- Worse around 9 p.m; between 3 a.m. and 4 a.m.; for **movement**; from becoming **hot**

- Better for lying on painful part; **hard pressure**, e.g. massage; open air; from rest; being quiet; **being still**

Eupatorium Perfoliatum

- Chill preceded by thirst and extreme **aching, deep in the bones**; intense back pain; feels **bruised** inside and out; severe headache with **pain at the back of head** when lying down; **sore eyeballs**; high **fever and chills alternate**; hoarseness, loose cough and **sore chest**; watery nasal discharge with sneezing; very **restless; craves cold food and drinks**

- Worse in open air; **between 7 a.m. and 9 a.m.**; for coughing; moving

- Better for sweating (except the headache); being indoors; being warmly covered; **getting on all fours**

Gelsemium

- Gradual onset; sensation of **heaviness** throughout body; fatigue, aching, **muscle weakness** and **soreness**; **trembling**; **drooping eyelids**; extreme **exhaustion**; fever with chills up and down spine; dizziness and **drowsiness**; dull headache, feels like a **tight band** around the head, above the eyes; thirstless

- Influenza from exposure to cold, damp weather; from **bad news**; from **anticipation**;

- Worse from anticipation (even of pleasurable events); **change of weather** (cold nights, warm days)

- Better for sweating; **urination**; in open air if not chilled; in the afternoon; **reclining** with head held high

Gelsemium is the number one flu remedy.

Nux Vomica

- High fever with sudden onset; body is burning hot, especially the face; very **chilly, must be covered up**; severe shivering or shaking; aching limbs and back; **gastric symptoms**, e.g. **nausea**, vomiting; loose stools; chill with thirst or heat without thirst; sour sweat, smells like musty straw; **hypersensitive** and **irritable**; hypochondria

- Influenza from exposure to cold east or northeast wind

- Worse with **cold draughts**; noise; light; touch; in the morning; in cold, dry weather

- Better with rest; hot drinks; **warmth**

Phos-ac

- **Exhaustion**; emotional and physical weakness; **dark circles** under eyes; **apathy** and **indifference**; sleepy by day; **brain fog**; lack of concentration; dizziness; **weak feeling in chest** from talking; dehydration; excess sweating; craves carbonated drinks and water-rich foods

- Use for **post-viral fatigue**

- Worse with strong emotions; when **talking** or being talked to; being cold; cold draughts

- Better after **short naps**; with warmth; in open air; **fizzy drinks**

Rhus Tox

- **Restlessness**; pain and **stiffness in lower back**; sore, aching limbs; discomfort when trying to rest; high fever but feels very cold as if **cold water runs through veins**; shivering if uncovered; **red tip of tongue**; craves cold milk, yogurt or cheese; anxiety and sadness

- Influenza from damp, cold weather; change in weather; getting **wet**; getting **chilled** from cold bathing

- Worse on waking; with the **cold**; with **dampness**; in the evening; being still; from ice-cold drinks

- Better **as the day goes on**; from **heat**; hot bathing; warm drinks; swallowing; movement; stretching; being wrapped up

OTHER HOME REMEDIES

Honey, lemon, ginger and garlic tonic

A blend of raw honey, lemon, ginger and garlic is a great way to ease the symptoms of flu and promote a speedy recovery. Well known for their health-restoring properties, these natural ingredients work together to strengthen the immune system and alleviate discomfort.

To soothe a sore throat and stop bacterial growth, add a tablespoon of raw honey to boiled water. Juice half a lemon for its vitamin C content, which helps break down mucus, then grate a thumbnail-sized piece of fresh ginger into the mixture for its anti-inflammatory benefits. For its immune-boosting properties, crush a clove of garlic and add to the mixture. Let the mixture steep for a few minutes and drink while it's still warm.

Turmeric 'golden milk'

The key component of turmeric is curcumin, which boasts antiviral, antibacterial and anti-inflammatory properties. For centuries, this vibrant yellow spice has been a cornerstone of Ayurvedic medicine.

Stir ¼ teaspoon of ground turmeric, a pinch of black pepper and a drizzle of oil (coconut, sesame, flax or ghee) into a glass of warm milk.

INSOMNIA

Insomnia is the term used to describe regular sleep disturbances. Rest is essential in helping the body to repair and recuperate, so long-term insomnia has repercussions on health and wellbeing. Many factors affect sleep quality, including stress, worry and depression.

Caring for young children, hormonal changes such as the menopause, as well as your environment – such as outside noise or hot, stuffy rooms – can also disturb sleep. Irregular sleep schedules due to shift work or jet lag will exacerbate the problem.

Signs of insomnia include

- Difficulty falling asleep and staying asleep
- Not getting back to sleep easily after waking in the night
- Waking up too early
- Waking up feeling unrefreshed and tired
- Poor focus and energy levels during the day
- Bad moods and irritability

Actions that may help:

- Exercise frequently.

- Maximize exposure to morning sunlight to support the circadian rhythm.

- Minimize exposure to blue-light screens in the evening.

- Avoid alcohol as it can disrupt the production of melatonin, the hormone that regulates sleep cycles.

- Reduce naps during the day.

- Be consistent with bedtimes and wake times.

- Create a conducive sleep environment.

- Avoid eating late in the evening.

- Try listening to a guided relaxation or meditation before you go to sleep.

HOMEOPATHIC REMEDIES

Arsenicum Album

- Wakes around **midnight** and can be awake until 3 a.m.; gets in and out of bed, walks around; anxiety on waking from frightful dreams; fear of being **alone** and **death**

- Sleeplessness from **anxiety**; **nervous exhaustion**; **restlessness**

- Worse around or after midnight; from lying on **right side**

- Better for company; heat; **motion**; warm drinks and food

Cocculus

- Mental or physical exhaustion; anxious and frightening dreams; sleep frequently disturbed by **fitful starts**; **fear of not getting enough sleep**; empty, **hollow feeling** in body, head, stomach, leg

- Sleeplessness from **thinking about work**; anxiety; restlessness; nursing loved ones; **night shifts**; **jet lag**

- Worse for loss of sleep; **nursing others**; noise; open air

- Better in a **warm room**; from lying quietly

Coffea Cruda

- Can't switch brain off, **rush of ideas**; **oversensitive nervous system**, all senses more acute; light sleeper, **woken by slightest sound**; great **agitation** and **restlessness**

- Sleeplessness from excessive consumption of **coffee** or wine; from **overexcitement** or overactive mental activity

- Worse with **noise**; **touch**; excitement; coffee; alcohol

- Better for rest; **lying down**

Ignatia

- Dreams about grief, death of loved ones or broken relationships; indecision and **conflicting ideas**; jerking limbs on falling asleep; **sleeps very lightly**, hears everything around them; frequently changes position in bed; **sighing** and whimpering while sleeping

- Sleeplessness due to **emotional conflict**, grief, disappointed love or **relationship worries**

- Worse for drinking **coffee**; **tobacco** smoke; strong emotions
- Better for **lying flat** on back; **deep breathing**

Kali Phos

- Feels very sensitive, **weak** and easily fatigued by the slightest thing; restlessness and **excess heat** during sleep; night terrors and **sleepwalking**
- Sleeplessness from overworking; excessive mental exertion; work/study worries; or **nervous insomnia** from **overactive mind**
- Worse from any mental and physical **exertion**
- Better for **warmth**; **rest**

Nux Vomica

- Unable to switch off from **work worries**; awakes with **fright** at the **slightest noise**, as if someone is in the room; awakes at 3 a.m. with a **rush of thoughts**, lies awake until morning; awakes feeling **unrefreshed** and nauseous; **busy**, anxious dreams; **needs alcohol** to wind down in the evening
- Sleeplessness from **mental strain**; excess of alcohol, **coffee** and **tobacco**
- Worse for alcohol; **working late**; eating **rich food**
- Better for **naps**; lying on **one side**; drinking **warm milk**

OTHER HOME REMEDIES

Chamomile tea with honey

Chamomile tea is celebrated for its calming effects and sleep-inducing properties. Add a small amount of honey to the chamomile tea to aid in relaxation and facilitate sleep. Honey contains trace amounts of tryptophan, an essential amino acid crucial for the production of serotonin and melatonin. These two chemicals are key players in regulating our sleep and relaxation cycles.

Lavender

Lavender is a natural remedy for insomnia due to its relaxing properties. Its scent is known to calm the nervous system and lower heart rate and blood pressure, creating an ideal state for sleep. It can significantly enhance sleep quality by promoting the deep, restorative stages of sleep. This results in a more peaceful night's rest and can be especially beneficial for individuals struggling to fall asleep.

Lavender can be used in various forms to promote better sleep, including aromatherapy using lavender essential oil, placing dried lavender sachets under the pillow or using lavender-infused bath products.

JET LAG

Flying, particularly a long-haul flight, can put strain on the body due to the lack of movement and the pressurized, recirculated air in the cabin. This environment can lead to dehydration because the air is low in humidity and can deplete the body's moisture levels. Drinking alcohol, coffee, tea and carbonated drinks during a flight may contribute to dehydration and worsen the symptoms of jet lag. Additionally, travelling across time zones, losing sleep, or staying up to adjust to a different time zone can significantly worsen jet lag.

Signs of jet lag include:

- General malaise and feeling out of sorts
- Sudden waves of tiredness
- Dizziness
- Digestive upsets including nausea, indigestion and/or constipation
- Difficulty concentrating
- Insomnia or disturbed sleep

Actions that may help:

- Stay hydrated by drinking plenty of fluids: approximately 300ml (10oz) of water every hour of the flight.

- Bring your own healthy snacks to eat on board.

- Get sun exposure to help regulate the body's internal clock.

- Take a short nap (20–30 minutes) during the day if you're excessively tired.

- Avoid caffeine, soft drinks and alcohol, especially near bedtime.

- Adjust your sleep schedule a few days before the trip by going to bed slightly earlier or later, depending on the direction of travel.

- Try to fast on a short flight. On a long flight, avoid eating at the time it would be your normal sleep time back home.

- Move around as much as possible during the flight. Every hour, try practising a deep-breathing exercise and doing 10 squats.

- Create a relaxing bedtime routine to help signal to the body that it's time to wind down.

HOMEOPATHIC REMEDIES

Arnica

This remedy is great for reducing the physical strain on the body of flying. It can help alleviate the feeling of being bruised or achy all over, which often occurs after long-haul flights. Taking arnica before and after a flight can noticeably reduce the overall sense of discomfort and malaise.

Cocculus

This remedy is particularly useful if jet lag is accompanied by mental and physical exhaustion from lack of sleep and time zone changes. Cocculus can help reset the body clock and is beneficial for symptoms like dizziness, difficulty concentrating and a hollow, empty feeling in the body. It's best to take Cocculus before the journey, during the flight and for a few days after arriving at the destination to help the body adjust.

MORNING SICKNESS

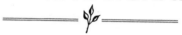

The term 'morning sickness' refers to the nausea and vomiting that commonly occur during the early stages of pregnancy. However, it's not just confined to the mornings; the severity of symptoms can vary greatly in each woman, and sometimes in each pregnancy, and can impact daily functions.

Morning sickness usually subsides between the 12th and 16th weeks of pregnancy and usually doesn't pose any risks to the baby. However, a more serious condition called Hyperemesis Gravidarum can be dangerous as it can lead to dehydration and malnourishment if not properly treated, and sometimes requires hospitalization.

If you experience severe or persistent symptoms, or if you struggle to keep food or fluids down, it's important to contact a healthcare practitioner for further guidance and treatment options.

Signs of morning sickness include:

- Nausea and/or vomiting, especially in the morning, although it can occur anytime of the day

- Increased sensitivity to certain smells

- Changes in appetite and a strong desire for or aversion to certain foods

Actions that may help:

- Eat small, frequent meals and drink sips of water throughout the day.

- Eat plain foods that are easy to digest, such as crackers, toast, rice and bananas.

- Get plenty of rest and relaxation.

HOMEOPATHIC REMEDIES

Cocculus

- **Nausea** with faintness and vomiting; nausea with **thought or sight of food and drink**; loss of appetite; **metallic taste** in mouth; retching and vomiting sour, bitter, foul-smelling discharge; **vertigo** and dizziness; thirst **without desire to drink**

- Worse from **lack of sleep**; exertion; motion sickness; **touch**; being too **cold**; eating cold food and drink

- Better for **sitting** or **lying quietly** in a warm room

Ipecac

- **Constant nausea and desire to vomit**, doesn't feel better afterwards; persistent vomiting; no appetite, disgust and loathing of all food; nausea from smell of food and looking at **moving objects**; **retching after drinking anything cold**; **profuse salivation**; sinking sensation in stomach; thirstless

- Worse for **warmth**; vomiting; **lying down**

- Better for rest; **closing eyes**; being in fresh, **open air**

Lactic Acid

- Nausea with **vomiting on waking**; **persistent nausea**, can last for days; feeling **seasick**; hot, **acrid belching**; **heartburn**; **copious salivation**; bad taste in mouth

- Worse from smelling tobacco smoke; on waking in the morning; **after breakfast**

- Better for **eating**; belching

Nux Vomica

- **Awakes with nausea** and sour taste in mouth; nausea, retching and vomiting; wants to vomit but can't; **headaches from stimulant withdrawal**, e.g. coffee, tea; **angry**; irritable; **impatient**; overactive mind; **very chilly**

- Worse with **cold**; **noise**; tight-fitting clothes around the **waist**

- Better for **naps**; warm drinks; after **vomiting**

Pulsatilla

- Pale face; feeling chilly; craves things that disagree later, e.g. pastry; **throbbing, right-sided headaches**; large appetite, followed by feeling overfull; **weepy**, emotional, anxious about being a good mother

- Worse in **stuffy rooms**; from eating hot food

- Better for cool, **open air**; having cold drinks

Sepia

- Aversion to sight, cooking, smell and thought of food; **hypersensitive to smells**; vomiting after eating; **nausea in the morning** before eating; faintness and weakness, not better after eating; feels chilly; **irritable**, **depressed**, weepy; **intolerant of loved ones**

- Worse on waking; when lying on **one side**; in cold air; from **strong odours**

- Better for **warmth**

Symphoricarpus

- **Extreme nausea**; aversion to and **disgust at smell and thought of all food**; bitter taste in mouth; **persistent vomiting**; **violent retching**

- Worse from odour of food; **any motion**; **on rising**

- Better when **lying on back**

OTHER HOME REMEDIES

Peppermint tea

Strong peppermint tea is an effective way to soothe the stomach and alleviate nausea and vomiting. When nauseous, sip this tea throughout the day.

Ginger tea

Ginger is a well-regarded home remedy for morning sickness due to its active components that have a soothing effect on digestion, helping to settle the nausea and vomiting of early pregnancy.

Slice or grate fresh ginger and steep in boiling water for several minutes, and drink throughout the day.

Lemon water

Lemon can help reduce feelings of nausea. Many pregnant women find that simply inhaling the fresh scent of a cut lemon can help alleviate symptoms of morning sickness. Drinking lemon water is a great way to manage nausea throughout the day and hydrate by replenishing fluids lost from regular vomiting.

To make lemon water, squeeze the juice of a fresh lemon into a glass of water. Adjust the amount of lemon to taste.

MOUTH ULCERS

Mouth ulcers are small sores that can appear on the lining of the mouth, gums or tongue. They are minor ailments that usually heal on their own within one to two weeks. Although not usually serious, they can be quite painful and make eating, drinking or talking difficult.

Mouth ulcers can be caused by hormonal changes, such as during pregnancy, or by deficiencies in vitamin B12 or iron. They can also have a genetic component, with some families being more prone to developing them than others. If you experience frequent mouth ulcers, seek guidance from a qualified healthcare practitioner.

Signs of mouth ulcers include:

- White, round and painful sores on the lining of the mouth or surface of the tongue and gums
- Pain when eating, drinking or brushing teeth
- Area around the ulcer can be red and inflamed
- Difficulty eating or speaking

Actions that may help:

- Use relaxation techniques or mediation to manage stress, which can exacerbate mouth ulcers.

- Avoid sugary or spicy foods, citrus fruits and tomatoes, as well as chewy or crunchy foods.

- Avoid acidic or carbonated drinks that may sting or aggravate the ulcers.

- Maintain good oral hygiene by using a soft toothbrush.

- Avoid tobacco and alcohol, as these can irritate ulcers and prevent healing.

- Apply a cold compress or ice to the affected area to reduce inflammation and pain.

HOMEOPATHIC REMEDIES

Arsenicum Album

- Mouth dryness and **burning heat**; bitter taste in mouth after eating and drinking; burning, **painful tongue**; swollen, bleeding gums; anxiety; **exhaustion**; **restlessness**

- Worse with **cold drinks and food**; on **right side**

- Better with **hot drinks**

Merc Sol

- **Very painful**, stinging ulcers; **metallic taste** in mouth; **increased saliva**; **foul-smelling breath**; great thirst for **cold drinks**; ulcers on gums and **tongue**; **difficulty speaking** due to pain

- Worse with **touch**; from **eating** food; at **night**

- Better in the **morning**

Nitric-ac

- Sharp, **splinter-like pains** from ulcers, often on soft palate; pimples on side of tongue; foul, putrid breath; bleeding tongue; excessive salivation, can **burn corners** of mouth; **angry**; **irritable**

- Ulcers from lack of sleep; from difficult life events, e.g. nursing a loved one, divorce; from side effects of medications

- Worse at **night**; with **touch**

- Better for **hot compresses**

OTHER HOME REMEDIES

Saltwater rinse

Dissolve a teaspoon of salt in a cup of warm water and rinse your mouth to disinfect the area and reduce inflammation.

Bicarbonate of soda

Make a paste from a teaspoon of bicarbonate of soda with a few drops of water to help neutralize acidity and reduce pain.

Honey

Due to its antibacterial properties, honey can be applied to the ulcer to promote healing and reduce the risk of infection.

Coconut oil

Known for its anti-inflammatory and antimicrobial properties, applying coconut oil to the ulcer can soothe the pain and reduce inflammation.

NOSEBLEEDS

A nosebleed happens when the small blood vessels in the nasal passages are broken. Some children are prone to nosebleeds, and they can occur spontaneously as they grow. A nosebleed can usually be managed at home and, although alarming, is not a serious health concern.

The most common causes of a nosebleed include a blow to the nose, excessive sneezing, breathing in harsh chemicals, high blood pressure and blood-thinning medications.

If the nosebleed persists for more than 20 to 30 minutes despite applying pressure, or if it's accompanied by other concerning symptoms such as dizziness, fainting or difficulty breathing, seek medical attention promptly.

Signs of nosebleeds include:

- Pressure or fullness sensation in the nose before a nosebleed
- Bleeding from one or both nostrils
- Blood may flow from the back of the nose down the throat
- Pink or red streaks on a tissue
- Warm or metallic taste in the mouth

Actions that may help:

- Stay calm – panicking can lead to an increase in heart rate and blood pressure, which may in turn cause increased bleeding.

- Sit in an upright position and tilt the head slightly forward. Do not lean back as this may cause choking by sending blood to the back of the throat.

- Use the thumb and index finger to pinch the soft part of the nose just below the bridge (above the nostrils) for five to 10 minutes, breathing through the mouth.

- Place an ice pack (wrapped in a cloth) or cold compress on the bridge of the nose or the back of the neck. The cold constricts the blood vessels of the nasal passages, reducing bleeding.

HOMEOPATHIC REMEDIES

These are the main homeopathic remedies that can be used as simple first aid solutions when dealing with nosebleeds.

Aconite

A reliable solution for sudden nosebleeds accompanied by panic, fear, anxiety and a numb sensation in the nose with bleeding.

Arnica

The first remedy to take following an accident or injury to the nose.

Ferrum Phos 6x

This is a common remedy for children who are prone to nosebleeds.

Phosphorous

A useful remedy, especially for young children or adults, when dealing with bright red bleeding that doesn't clot easily and can result from the slightest activity, such as blowing the nose.

OTHER HOME REMEDIES

Apple cider vinegar

Apple cider vinegar causes the blood vessels to constrict, reducing blood flow. Soak a cotton wool ball with apple cider vinegar and gently place it in the affected nostril for 10 minutes.

Cayenne pepper

Cayenne pepper stimulates blood clotting and can help to stem bleeding. For a nosebleed, mix a small amount of cayenne pepper powder into warm water and drink it. This remedy works surprisingly quickly.

PERIOD PAIN

Period pain is a common complaint that most women will experience at some point in their menstruating life. It varies in intensity and duration and can change from one period to the next. For some women, it's very debilitating, and they find it difficult to function for a few days.

Signs of period pain include:

- Discomfort before and during a period, with pain a few days before and for a few days after

- Persistent dull ache in the lower abdomen

- Spasmodic cramping pain: mild or severe in the lower abdomen

- Pelvic pain that radiates and travels into the lower back or thighs

Actions that may help:

- A hot water bottle, heat pad or warm bath can relax the muscles and give some relief.

- Gentle, light exercise such as walking or stretching can help increase blood flow and release endorphins, the body's natural painkillers.

- Ease the pain in the abdomen or back with gentle massage.

- Prioritize rest and sleep.

HOMEOPATHIC REMEDIES

Belladonna

- Menstrual cramps **during period**; feelings of heaviness around lower abdomen; **fast**, intense, **throbbing**, sharp, **sudden pain** that comes in waves; profuse, **bright red** bleeding; sensitive to draughts, desire to be wrapped up warmly

- Worse for **lying down**; being overly hot; between **3 p.m. and 9 p.m.**

- Better for standing; **sitting upright**; bending backwards

Caulophyllum

- Severe **labour-like** pain; **irregular** period (since **puberty**); pain in **thigh**, as if muscles have been pulled; **shooting, cramping** pains with **nausea**, vomiting and pain in **lumbar region before period starts**; feels very **tired** and heavy; pain in **small joints**, especially fingers and toes, before period starts; spotting and bleeding between periods

- Worse in open air; from drinking **coffee**; with **motion**

- Better for **warmth**; once period starts

Chamomilla

- Labour-like period pain with brown blood and clots; very **angry** and **irritable**; **oversensitive** to pain; **impulsive**; **cutting pain** that runs up and down **inner thighs**

- Worse at night; from drinking coffee; with **strong emotions**

- Better for **cold applications**; vigorous **walking**

Cimicifuga

- Severe pain, **gets worse as flow gets heavier**; cramping, sharp, shooting pain, like **electric shocks**; backache and muscle spasms during period; **sharp pain from hip to hip** or shooting into thighs; **depression**; irregular periods

- Worse for drinking **wine**; **draughts**; sitting; heat; at **night**

- Better in **open air**; from being warmly **wrapped up**

Colocynthis

- **Intense**, **gripping**, **cramping pain**; needs to **bend double, roll up in a ball** or draw knees to chest to relieve the pain; **sudden** and **violent** pains, may cause individual to **cry out** or **vomit**; pain focused on **left side** of body; very **angry** and irritable

- Worse from being cold; **suppressed emotions**; lying on the painless side

- Better for warmth; **lying on abdomen**; bending over

Mag Phos

- Severe menstrual cramps with **radiating** pains; **sudden, shooting pains** like lightning or a **pressing pain** with a sense of constriction; pain at night **before period starts**; pain focused on **right side** of body; sweating; **anxiety**

- Worse from **cold air**; touch; **exertion**

- Better for **rubbing**; **warm applications**; heat; rest; hard pressure; bending double

Pulsatilla

- **Erratic** periods, **changeable** from month to month; changeable menstrual flow, e.g. heavier during the day and when walking; painful periods **since puberty**; **weepy** before period starts, craves **affection** and sympathy, can feel **abandoned**; intense bearing-down pains; **cold, pale face** during period; diarrhoea; **thirstless**

- Worse in **warm, stuffy rooms**; from **lying down**

- Better in **cool, open air**; being consoled; with massage; **cold applications**

Sepia

- Painful, irregular period that often arrives early; **light flow**; **bloating** and **low energy** before period starts; craves chocolate; **dragging, bearing-down sensation**; very **irritable**; sensitive; desires **solitude**; **intolerant** of loved ones

- Linked to **hormonal changes**: puberty, childbirth, after weaning, contraceptive pill

- Worse from cold air; in morning and evening; from **standing**

- Better with **physical activity** and exercise; in warm bed; **being busy**

OTHER HOME REMEDIES

Ginger tea

Ginger is a natural anti-inflammatory and can soothe menstrual cramps. Boiling fresh ginger slices in water and drinking this tea throughout the day can help lessen the intensity of period pain.

Chamomile tea

Drinking chamomile tea can help soothe menstrual cramps. Its antispasmodic effects calm and relax the body and ease period pain. Chamomile also helps with sleep regulation and mood, so it can help you feel more like your normal self.

Epsom salts bath

Epsom salts are a magnesium compound that can ease the cramping and pain of a period and boost magnesium uptake. Add one or two cups of Epsom salts to a bath and stir the water until the salts are fully dissolved. Soak in the bath for at least 20 minutes to maximize the effects of the magnesium salts.

PREMENSTRUAL SYNDROME (PMS)

Premenstrual syndrome (PMS) is a collection of symptoms that some women experience before their menstrual period. These can be a mental, emotional and physical and last anywhere from a few days to two weeks leading up to their period.

Signs of PMS include:

- Mood swings, irritability and depression
- Feeling out of control with angry outbursts or crying
- Enlargement or tenderness of the breasts
- Low energy
- Bloating and fluid retention
- Spotty skin and greasy hair
- Headaches

Actions that may help:

- Sleep well.
- Engage in physical activity or exercise.

- Avoid salty foods, which may cause fluid retention.

- Avoid caffeine and alcohol.

- Eat little and often to avoid bloating.

- Keep a journal to record moods and feelings throughout the month.

- Eat a healthy, balanced diet that provides sufficient magnesium and B vitamins, especially B6 and B12.

HOMEOPATHIC REMEDIES

Lachesis

- **Jealous**; **suspicious**; angry; **vengeful**; paranoid, feels persecuted; **talkative**; depression; headaches; fluid retention; weight gain; symptoms focused on **left side** of body

- Linked to **hormonal changes**: puberty, childbirth, weaning, contraceptive pill

- Worse after **sleep**; with **heat**; **alcohol**; **pressure** from tight-fitting clothes around waist or neck

- Better **after period starts**; in open air

Lycopodium

- Wants to be alone, but have **someone close by** in the next room; indecisive; **lacks confidence**; **low self-esteem**; irritable; **domineering** to family members; **ravenous** appetite; craves sweets; **bloated** abdomen after eating, even a **small amount**; right-sided **headaches**; depression; **indigestion**

- Worse on **right side**; in a warm room; on waking; from tight-fitting clothes; when taking the **contraceptive pill**

- Better for consuming **warm food and drinks**; with **motion**

Natrum Mur

- **Withdrawn**; emotionally **shut down**; **dwells on the past**; **sad**; easily offended; cold sores on lips; **aversion to sex**; **fluid retention**; cold hands and feet; **constipation**; dry, hard stools; strong **thirst**; **craves salt**

- Worse with **sympathy**; **consolation**; between sunrise to sunset

- Better in open air; with tight clothing; rest; **being alone**

Pulsatilla

- **Erratic** periods, **changeable** from month to month; **weepy**; craves **affection** and sympathy; feels **abandoned** and unlovable; changeable moods; **very sensitive** to what others say; changeable, shifting symptoms; **thirstless**

- Linked to **hormonal changes**: puberty, childbirth, weaning, contraceptive pill

- Worse in **warm**, **stuffy rooms**; from lying down

- Better for cool, fresh, **open air**; with **consolation**; massage; **cold applications**

Sepia

- Very **irritable**; **exhausted**; emotionally flat, **indifferent** but will sometimes cry; desires solitude; **intolerant** of loved ones; **loss of libido**; swollen, **sensitive breasts**; spots or **acne**

- Linked to **hormonal changes**: puberty, childbirth, weaning, contraceptive pill

- Worse in **cold air**; morning and evening; from **standing**

- Better for **physical activity** and exercise

OTHER HOME REMEDIES

Peppermint tea

Drinking peppermint tea can help relieve bloating and any other digestive problems associated with PMS.

Chamomile tea

Chamomile can help soothe and relax the body, reducing stress, anxiety and irritability. It also helps with sleep and mood regulation for overall wellbeing.

SHOCK (EMOTIONAL)

Emotional shock is a strong reaction to a distressing event or news. It can lead to lasting emotions such as anxiety, fright, post-traumatic stress, anger outbursts, depression, sleep disturbance and loss of appetite. Emotional shock can also cause distress, excessive crying, loss of confidence and may take time to recover from. Taking homeopathic remedies can help prevent shock from turning into a long-held trauma.

Healing from emotional shock takes time, patience and kindness. If symptoms persist (more than 6–8 weeks) and become overwhelming, seek advice from a qualified healthcare professional.

Signs of shock include:

- Feelings of detachment or numbness
- Intense fear or anxiety
- Confusion or disorientation
- Denial or disbelief
- Feeling overwhelmed
- Emotional outbursts

- Shaking, trembling, rapid heartbeat, nausea or dizziness

- Flashbacks

- Sleep disturbances

Actions that may help:

- Talk to someone: a trusted family member, friend or therapist.

- Try a deep-breathing exercise: inhale deeply through the nose and exhale slowly through the mouth.

- Take time out for yourself, to nurture and focus on your wellbeing, e.g. go for a massage or take a relaxing bath.

- Establish a routine as soon as possible and plan your time.

HOMEOPATHIC REMEDIES

Aconite

- **Very anxious** and **fearful**; distressed; prone to **panic attacks**; staring, **glassy eyes**; dilated pupils; fear of impending death; physical or mental **restlessness**

- Emotional shock from a **fright**

- Worse at **night** (around midnight)

- Better in **open air**

Arnica

- **Confusion**; drowsiness; struggles to express themselves; **underestimates severity** of situation, declines help; wants to be alone; **fear of being approached** by anyone

- Emotional shock from a **physical trauma or injury**, e.g. fall or blow

- Worse for **touch**; in the evening; at night

- Better for **lying down**; being outstretched

Gelsemium

- Anxiety; confusion; **apathy**; dizziness; **drowsiness**; physical **weakness**; **trembling**; sleepiness; dilated pupils and **droopy eyelids**; desires **solitude** and quiet

- Emotional shock from receiving **bad news**

- Worse with **tobacco smoking**

- Better for walking; **physical movement**

Ignatia

- Distressed; **tearful**; **highly emotional** with outbursts of **sobbing**; **controlled**, tries to keep emotion in with **deep sighing**; oversensitive; **mood swings**; sensation of **lump in throat**; insomnia

- Emotional shock after losing a loved one or object with a deep emotional attachment; or from significant **disappointment**

- Worse for **consolation**; **coffee**; tobacco smoking; stimulants

- Better for swallowing; pressure; **being alone**

OTHER HOME REMEDIES

Rescue Remedy

Rescue Remedy is a blend of 5 Bach flower remedies that can help to calm the nervous system and alleviate distress following an emotional shock.

To use, place four drops of Rescue Remedy directly on the tongue or add four drops to water and sip at intervals. Repeat as needed.

SORE THROATS

A sore throat is often the first symptom of a cold or flu, signalling the body is unwell. The tonsils are believed to act as a first line of defence in the immune system, helping to prevent a common cold turning into a more serious issue, such as a chest infection. Typically, a sore throat goes away within a few days. If symptoms persist or worsen, and are accompanied by difficulty breathing or swallowing, seek medical help.

Signs of sore throat include:

- Pain or soreness in the throat, worse when swallowing
- Dry, scratchy throat
- Back of the mouth looks red and inflamed
- Smelly breath
- Swollen glands in the neck or behind the ears

Actions that may help:

- Suck on an ice cube if it eases the pain.
- Sip warm drinks if the pain is better for heat.
- Try a steam inhalation (see page 72).
- Get more sleep and rest.

HOMEOPATHIC REMEDIES

Aconite

- **Sudden onset**; acute inflammation of throat with high fever; **red, dry, hot, burning throat** with stinging or pricking pain; **constricted feeling**, inability to swallow; choking on swallowing; hoarseness with pain when talking; restlessness, especially at night; **anxiety**; very thirsty for cold drinks

- Sore throat from exposure to **dry, cold winds**; from getting very cold; after a **shock** or **fright**

- Worse at **midnight**; with touch; **swallowing**

- Better with **rest**; from **not talking**

Belladonna

- Sudden onset; **high fever**; **swollen glands**; **angry, red** throat, **looks glossy**; **right-sided throbbing pain**, can extend to ears when swallowing; **dry, hot** throat; throat feels **constricted**, sensation of lump in throat; red and bumpy '**strawberry tongue**'; thirsty but difficulty swallowing liquids; flushed, red face or very pale

- Sore throat from exposure to **dry, cold winds**; from getting very cold; from head getting wet; after a **shock** or **fright**; sore throats in **children**

- Worse with **slightest touch to throat**; turning head; **swallowing liquids**

- Better when **eating solid food**; drinking

Hepar Sulph

- **Splinter-like pains** in the throat, sensation of stuck, **sharp fish bone**; pain can **extend to ears** when swallowing; **very chilly** and sensitive to cold; thick, **stringy, yellow mucus** in throat, constant need to cough it up; very **irritable** and **oversensitive**

- Worse with **touch**; anything **cold**

- Better with **warm applications**; **warm drinks**; being wrapped up

Lachesis

- Pain starts on **left side** of throat but can move to right side; very painful, **can't bear anything touching the neck**; swollen, **constricted** feeling, like lump in throat; **purple or bluish tonsils**

- Worse with **hot drinks**; when **swallowing liquids** (even saliva); with **slight pressure on neck**; on waking

- Better for **cold drinks**; **swallowing solid food**

Lycopodium

- Stitch-like pain begins on **right-hand side** but will often **move to left side**; dryness of throat **without thirst**; sharp pains on swallowing; **sensation of ball ascending in throat**; foul breath; enlargement of tonsils and **ulceration**

- Worse with **cold drinks**; between 4 p.m. and 8 p.m; after sleep

- Better for **warm drinks and food**

Merc Sol

- **Right-sided**, raw, **burning** pain in throat, **extends to ears** on swallowing; swollen, painful glands; sensation of **hot vapour rising** or **apple core stuck** in throat; **putrid breath**; **excessive salivation**; **yellow tongue**; **metallic taste** in mouth; dry throat with constant **desire to swallow**; enlarged tonsils and ulceration; profuse, **smelly sweat** at night; difficulty speaking; anxiety; very thirsty for cold drinks

- Individuals with a history of sore throat, with many courses of antibiotics

- Worse with **heat or cold**; touch; empty swallowing; **change in weather**; coughing; at **night**

- Better for **lying down**

Phytolacca

- **Right-sided** burning pain; **swollen, tender glands**; **stiff neck**; **dry**, **rough**, very **hot**, constricted throat; **dark red**, hot, swollen tonsils; **back of tongue feels scalded** or burnt; **shooting pains into ears** on swallowing; **restlessness**

- For chronic sore throat

- Worse from **swallowing**; **hot drinks**; exposure to **damp, cold weather**; movement

- Better for **warm, dry weather**; with **cold drinks**; rest

Rhus Tox

- Hoarseness; red, puffy throat; **itching in back of throat**; stinging pain in tonsils; **pain begins on left and moves to right side**; difficulty swallowing solids; **stiff throat and neck muscles**; dry throat and tongue; **red tip of tongue**; **restlessness**

- Sore throat from overusing or **straining the voice**, or from damp weather

- Worse **on waking**; from **talking**; eating

- Better **as the day goes on**; from **heat**; warm drinks; swallowing; movement

OTHER HOME REMEDIES

Honey and lemon tea

Honey has many health benefits and is often a key ingredient in sore throat remedies. Raw honey is more desirable as it hasn't been heated. With its antimicrobial properties and thick texture, it coats the throat, helping to ease the soreness and relieve inflamed areas. The lemon adds a dose of vitamin C, essential for immune defence. Squeeze half a lemon into boiled water and add a spoonful of honey to make a tea to drink throughout the day.

Garlic

Garlic contains allicin, which kills bacterial, fungal and viral growth. It can be very helpful for sore throats but is best taken raw. To make it more palatable, crush a garlic clove and add it to apple juice, or honey and lemon tea.

Saltwater gargle

Saltwater gargling can help ease the pain of a sore throat and kill bacteria and other microbes. To do this, dissolve half a teaspoon of salt in a cup of warm water, gargle with the solution, and then spit it out. Repeat this process two to three times a day. This remedy is not recommended for young children, who may swallow the mixture instead of gargling.

STRAINS AND SPRAINS

Strains and sprains affect different tissues but often occur in the same areas of the body. They refer to injuries that usually follow physical activity. A strain is an injury to a muscle or tendon, sometimes caused by repetitive action, and a sprain is caused by overstretching or tearing ligaments that hold two bones together, i.e. joints. Strains can happen suddenly in the case of a tear. A severe tear from a strain or sprain might need surgery, so seek medical advice if there is excessive swelling and pain or no improvement.

Signs of a strain include:

- Cramping pain and swelling

- Muscle spasms and muscle weakness

- A 'pop' feeling when the injury happens

Sprains are mostly seen in ankles, knees or wrists. Signs of a sprain include:

- Pain, swelling and bruising

- Inability to move or put weight on the affected joint

- A 'snap' sound when the injury happens

Actions that may help:

- For a less severe injury, follow the RICE method (Rest, Ice, Compression and Elevation) to help reduce swelling and pain.

- Take time to recover and move the affected area appropriately.

HOMEOPATHIC REMEDIES

Arnica

- **Sore**, **swollen**, **bruised** soft tissues around the joint; fear of touch or being examined

- Muscle or tendon injury after **prolonged or unaccustomed exertion**

- Worse for **touch**; applied pressure; the cold

- Better for rest; **lying down**

Arnica is the first remedy to give immediately after an injury occurs.

Bellis Perennis

- Intense pain; **soreness**; **aching**; **bruising**; **stiffness**

- Useful for **deeper soft tissue injuries**; after **overworking** a muscle or joint; for repetitive strain injuries

- Worse for **cold bathing**; touch; exertion

- Better with **heat application**

Bellis Perennis is a good alternative to Arnica and Ruta Grav as it addresses both joint weakness and a lame feeling, together with bruising and soreness – it's a good in-between.

Bryonia

- Affected area is **red** and **hot**; **sharp pain** during any movement; **stiffness** with painful **swelling**; **irritable**; wants to be left alone

- For strained and pulled **muscles**; sprained or injured **joints**

- Worse with **movement**; touch; **lying on unaffected side**

- Better for **being still**; cold applications; **compression**; **lying on affected side**

Rhus Tox

- **Shooting, tearing, stitch-like** pains; **stiffness**; **restlessness**

- Injuries from **overuse**; strain injuries from **heavy lifting**; tendons, ligaments, tissues

- Worse during **first movement**; from **being still**; sitting; at **night**

- Better with **continued movement**; **applied heat**; hot baths; massage; stretching

Ruta Grav

- **Soreness**; **aching**; **restlessness**; sharp, **shooting pains**; stiffness

- Use for injuries to tendons, joints and bones; **severe sprains** where there is a bruised bone, torn tendon or split ligament; recent or old injuries to knees or elbows; **repetitive strain injury,** e.g. tennis elbow or carpal tunnel syndrome; **eye strain** with headaches from reading fine print or carrying out detailed work

- Worse from **cold**; **dampness**; exertion; lying on affected part

- Better for **warmth**; heat application; **gentle motion**; rubbing

Strontium Carb

- **Swollen** ankles; ice-cold feet; chronic **spasms of ankle joint**; leg and foot cramps

- Use for chronic, **repeated sprains** of the ankles

- Worse with **cold**; touch; walking

- Better for immersing in **hot water**

OTHER HOME REMEDIES

Frankincense and peppermint oil

To help with inflammation and bruising, massage with a blend of frankincense and peppermint oils. Add a few drops of each essential oil to a carrier oil such as almond, coconut or olive oil. Rub the mixture gently into the affected area three times a day. Placing a warm cloth on the affected area afterwards can help with absorption and ease discomfort.

Castor oil

Castor oil has been recognized for its healing properties for centuries and can help to reduce inflammation from a strain or sprain. To apply, warm up the castor oil and massage onto the injured area, then cover it with a warm cloth or towel to aid absorption. If the pain allows, apply a hot water bottle or hot pad for 20–30 minutes to increase blood flow to the area and maximize the therapeutic effects of the oil. Wash off any leftover residue.

STYES

A stye is commonly caused by bacteria infecting an eyelash follicle or eyelid gland. It appears as a red or white lump on the eyelid that can be tender to the touch. There may be crusting around the stye and an increase in tears or discharge from the affected eye. Styes can be common in children.

It's important to avoid squeezing or popping the stye as this can make it worse. A style typically resolves in 10 to 14 days but can be very irritating. If it doesn't go away on its own, becomes worse or recurs frequently, it's advisable to see a professional practitioner for additional treatment.

Signs of styes include:

- Affected area can be red and inflamed

- Red or white swelling or lump on the eyelid

- Lump can be tender to the touch

- Irritation and pain on the affected eye

- Watering of the eye

- Crusting around the eye margin with yellow discharge

- Worse on waking in the morning

Actions that may help:

- Keep the affected area clean and gently remove any crusts or discharge.

- Do not rub or squeeze the stye.

- Wash hands regularly and use separate towels.

- Avoid wearing contact lenses or eye makeup as they can cause further irritation.

HOMEOPATHIC REMEDIES

Argent Nit

- **Red, swollen** eye, looks like **raw beef**, sensitive to light; **smelly, creamy, yellow discharge**; eyelids glued together with thick crusts; red, swollen, **inflamed** inner corners of eyes and eyelids; aching, tired eyes; **anxiety**; apprehension; **craves sugar**

- Worse in a **warm room**; in **left eye**

- Better for **cold compress**; pressure; closing eyes; with cool air

Graphites

- **Red, dry, swollen, sore, cracked eyelid**; styes on **lower lid** with **drawing pain**; thin, acrid discharge or **sticky, honey-like discharge** on eyelids on waking

- Worse for **daylight**; artificial light

- Better for open air; in **darkness**

Hepar Sulph

- Red, swollen, inflamed eyelid, **very sensitive to touch** and cold air; **splinter-like feeling** in the eye, grainy or sandy feeling; inflamed with **thick, yellow discharge**; **oversensitive**; **irritable**

- Worse with the **slightest draught**; in open air; with touch; **cold**; on waking

- Better for **warmth**; warm applications

Pulsatilla

- **Inflamed eyelid**, usually **upper left lid**; **eyelids stuck together**; profuse, **thick, yellow discharge** from infected eye; burning, itching eyes; **weepy, emotional**; changeable symptoms

- Worse in the morning; **on waking**

- Better with company; **sympathy**; **cold applications**; in **open air**

Staphysagria

- **Recurring styes**, often on left upper eyelid; no pus; **hard nodule or lump**; **pain in upper lid**, difficulty closing eye; **dry**, itchy eye, usually the left, very **sensitive**; hot tears

- Styes cause by **suppressed emotions**, especially **humiliation** and **anger**

- Worse when eye is **closed**; with **touch**; from suppressed emotions

- Better with a **cold compress**

Sulphur

- **Recurring styes in same place**, typically on **upper lids**; red, hot, stinging, burning, **itching eyelid margin**; profuse flow of oily tears with **burning** sensation; eyelids stuck together in morning with yellow or whitish discharge; **dry** eyes in warm room, but tears flow in open air
- Worse in the **morning**; when **bathing** the eye; in a stuffy room
- Better in **open air**

OTHER HOME REMEDIES

Warm compress

Applying a warm compress to the eyelid a few times a day can help in draining the stye.

Hypericum and Calendula herbal tincture (Hyper Cal)

This useful tincture combines Marigold and St John's Wort, which together act as an antiseptic, soothing the eye and reducing the swelling.

Boil some water and wait for it to cool down enough to use. Add a few drops of the tincture to the warm water, then soak a clean cloth and hold it against the affected eye for five minutes. Repeat this process for three or four times a day.

Chamomile tea

Chamomile can soothe the redness and soreness of a stye. Use a warm, wet tea bag as an eye compress, or make the tea and leave it to cool down to a warm temperature before soaking a cotton wool pad or clean cloth. Hold the pad against the stye for five minutes.

SUNSTROKE
(HEATSTROKE)

Sunstroke, also known as heatstroke, occurs when the body becomes overheated and is unable to cool down through its normal sweating mechanism. The body remains excessively hot, and the additional heat can lead to organ damage. Sunstroke typically occurs in hot climates or during heatwaves and is considered a serious emergency requiring immediate attention. Heat exhaustion, which precedes heatstroke, is not life-threatening but shares similar symptoms.

Signs of sunstroke and heatstroke include:

- Skin is pale and clammy, or dry and hot

- Dizziness, confusion and drowsiness

- Excessive sweating

- Raised body temperature

- Rapid heart rate and breathing

- Headache

- Nausea and or vomiting

- Excessive thirst

Actions that may help:

- Get out of the heat and act quickly to cool down the body.

- Place a cold, wet cloth or ice pack wrapped in a cloth under the armpits, in the groin and around the neck.

- Use cold, wet towels to cover the body or have a cold bath or cold shower, whichever method is quickest.

- Hydration is crucial and it's important to replace the electrolytes lost in the process of overheating. Consider taking rehydration salts.

HOMEOPATHIC REMEDIES

These acute remedies can be effective for mild cases of sunstroke or heatstroke. They should not be used in severe cases. The condition may need to be monitored so seek professional help.

Belladonna

- **Sudden onset**; **hot**, **red face**; congestion headache, forehead feels swollen; **throbbing**, **right-sided** pain in temples; pounding head on standing up; symptoms start around **late afternoon** and continue into night; **craves lemons** and lemonade; thirsty for cold water

- Worse for noise; **light**; **jarring motion**

- Better for applying **pressure** to the head; from **bending the head backwards**

Glonoine

- **Flushed face**; **splitting headache**; full, **bursting** feeling in head; waves of **pounding** pain; sits with **head in hands**, keeping head as still as possible; **throbbing** in temples; **flashes of light** before eyes

- Worse with walking; heat; movement; sun exposure; **lying down**

- Better for **elevating head**; cold applications; **being still**

Natrum Mur

- Bursting, **blinding headache**; **pain over eyes** and top of head; visual disturbances and **sensitivity to light**; tiredness and **weakness**; blotchy or **hive-like rash** that itches and burns; strong thirst; **craves salt**

- Worse on **waking**; from sunrise to sunset

- Better with **sleep**; pressure; lying with **head held high**; sitting still

OTHER HOME REMEDIES

Natural rehydration drink

Fluid loss can occur from excessive sweating, vomiting, bouts of diarrhoea and overheating. To stay hydrated or to rebalance hydration during illness or after physical activity, prepare a rehydration drink.

To make a rehydration drink, mix the following ingredients:

- 2 cups of water

- Juice from half a lemon

- ⅛ teaspoon of Celtic sea salt

- ¼ teaspoon to 1 tablespoon of a natural sweetener (options include honey, agave syrup or maple syrup)

Lemons

Lemons are rich in essential nutrients that support good hydration. Lemonade is an age-old traditional remedy used by people living in hot climates to stay hydrated.

TEETHING

Teething refers to the process of infant teeth breaking through the gums. The teething experience can vary; some children are born with their baby teeth, while others may not have visible teeth until 12 months of age. Typically, teeth appear around six months, but symptoms can begin as early as four months. Not all emerging teeth cause pain. By the time children are three years old, they usually have a full set of first teeth.

Signs of teething include:

- Gums look red and sore
- Mild fever
- One cheek is red or a rash develops on one side of the face
- Rubbing or pulling the ear
- Drooling, an increase of saliva
- Biting on things
- Being clingy, fretful or irritable, difficult to calm
- Sleep disturbance
- Stools change in colour

Actions that may help:

- Rub or massage the baby's gums with a clean finger.
- Use a wooden spoon cooled in the fridge for the baby to press their gums on.
- Comfort the baby with hugs and cuddles.
- Try to maintain a regular sleep routine, as teething can disrupt sleep patterns.

HOMEOPATHIC REMEDIES

Belladonna

- **Hot, red gums**; **fast**, sudden **intense** pains, especially lower teeth on **right side**; red, **dry, burning hot cheeks**; **high fever**; **glassy eyes**; **dilated pupils**; thirstless; **very sensitive** to touch; all senses heightened
- Worse at **night**; when eating; with **touch**; jarring motion
- Better when **biting on something**

Calc Carb

- Makes chewing motions and presses gums together; **shy** or reserved in new situations; plays independently without fuss; **sweats easily at night**, especially on **head**, leaves pillow damp and sour-smelling; **nightmares** or terrors; large appetite; **sour-smelling diarrhoea**; thirsty for cold drinks
- Good remedy for children with **slow, difficult** or **delayed teething**

- Worse in **cold, open air**; with milk; **hot food**
- Better after breakfast; with soothing from **touch**

Chamomilla

- Intolerable pain; highly **emotional**; **oversensitive**; temperamental; **irritable**; **angry**; restlessness; tantrums; **one cheek red** where tooth is coming through, **the other pale**; diarrhoea with **grass-green stools** like chopped eggs and spinach; thirsty for **cold drinks**
- Worse for touch; being looked at; **between 9 p.m. and midnight**; when cold; with **warm drinks**
- Better for being **carried**; with **cold applications**

Mag Phos

- **Hypersensitive** to pain; shouting or screaming; **restlessness**; **nervous**; sobbing; **despair**; **anxiety**; fear of being touched; exhaustion
- Worse for **cold water**; at night; with **light touch**; motion; in cold air
- Better for **heat** and warmth; **chewing on something hard**; rubbing

If Chamomilla doesn't work, try Mag Phos.

Pulsatilla

- **Yellow-green nasal discharge**; very **tearful** and **clingy**; wants to be **held** and **carried** everywhere; **thirstless**
- Worse in **stuffy rooms**; after sunset; from heat of bed coverings
- Better for **open air**; **cold applications**; being carried; **consolation**

Calc Phos 6x

Calc Phos is a vital remedy for growth and development, particularly influencing the nutrition of bones and teeth. This cell salt works on the inner structure of the teeth and is an excellent remedy for supporting the development of children's bones and teeth. It's especially beneficial for slow and difficult teething or when teething is delayed. Calc Phos also aids in resolving issues with teeth cutting through the gums. Furthermore, it's a good remedy for teeth that tend to decay early.

OTHER HOME REMEDIES

Homemade teething cream

Melt coconut oil and food-grade cocoa butter together and then mix in a few drops of clove oil. Be careful not to add too much clove oil, as it can be irritating and has a strong taste. Allow the mixture to set in the fridge. Once solid, apply it to the gums.

Chilled washcloths

Use clean, fresh drinking water to soak a washcloth. Put the wet washcloth in the freezer for an hour. Once it's cold but not too frozen to hold, the baby can suck on it.

Chamomile tea

Chamomile can help soothe sore gums. Soak a washcloth in cold chamomile tea and chill in the freezer, then allow the baby to suck on it.

TOOTH ABSCESS

A tooth abscess is a bacterial infection that results in the formation and build-up of pus. This pus can become trapped, causing pressure and pain. A tooth abscess often occurs from tooth decay but can also arise after a tooth is chipped or broken, or when dental work becomes infected.

A dental abscess requires professional treatment, including drainage of the abscess. If you suspect you have a tooth abscess, schedule an appointment with a dentist as soon as possible.

The signs of a tooth abscess include:

- Severe, persistent, throbbing toothache
- Pain radiating from the jawbone to the ears and neck
- Pain from contact with hot and cold
- Pain when chewing or biting
- Fever
- Swelling of the face at the site of the infected tooth
- Tender or swollen glands
- Foul-smelling, foul-tasting, salty fluid in the mouth

Actions that may help:

- A cold compress or ice pack wrapped in a cloth applied externally to the affected area may ease the pain and swelling.

- When in bed, elevate the head to help reduce blood flow to the painful area and alleviate pressure on the tooth.

- Avoid hot or cold food or drink that may trigger the pain.

- Maintain good oral hygiene to keep the affected tooth clean and free of debris.

HOMEOPATHIC REMEDIES

Belladonna

- Early-stage infection; **sudden**, violent, **throbbing** and shooting pain, comes and goes; dry mouth; sensation of **fullness** and **swelling** in affected part; throbbing pain in head; hot, red face

- Worse with **heat**; **jarring motion**; **touch**; **lying down**

- Better when **biting** on something; **leaning head** against something

Hepar Sulph

- Very **painful, sensitive**, pus-filled abscess; **splinter-like pain**; **very chilly**; very irritable

- Worse for lying on affected part; with **touch**; **cold draughts** or wind

- Better for **heat**

Silica

- Abscess at **root** of tooth; sensitive to **cold water** and **cold air**; foul-smelling **pus**
- Worse with **touch**; cold
- Better for **warmth**

OTHER HOME REMEDIES

Saltwater rinse

Saltwater rinses have antibacterial and healing properties and help draw out the pus, releasing some pressure from the abscess. To make a rinse, add one teaspoon of salt (if too tender, use half a teaspoon) to a glass of warm boiled water, then stir. Rinse the mouth with the saltwater every couple of hours.

Coconut oil rinse

With its antimicrobial properties, coconut oil may help protect against harmful bacteria. An oil rinse has been found to keep gums healthy and reduce plaque build-up, preventing gingivitis, bad breath and tooth decay. Daily practice is recommended for optimum results, morning and night before eating or drinking.

Take one tablespoon of coconut oil, preferably a food-grade, cold-pressed organic oil. Melt the oil in your mouth and swish it around your teeth for 10 minutes. Spit the oil out into a bin (not into a sink or toilet, as once cold, the oil will harden and clog up the water pipes). Don't swallow the oil as it contains bacteria and toxins from the mouth. Rinse out the mouth with water.

TOOTHACHES

Toothache can result from tooth decay, gum disease or an abscess and can be extremely painful. If you have a persistent toothache or an abscess, seek help from a dentist.

Tooth decay is the main cause of toothaches. The pain begins when the decay has eroded the hard enamel layer of the tooth and reached the dentin, a softer layer that protects the nerves. The decay progresses rapidly and causes pain once it reaches the dentin.

Gum infection or disease is inflammation of the gums. It can cause soreness and tooth pain. An infection in the gums can reach the tooth's root or the jawbone, causing intense pain.

An abscess forms when the infection reaches the middle layer of the tooth known as the pulp. Pus develops in a pocket, causing severe throbbing pain, a mild fever and a feeling of being unwell.

Signs of toothache include:

- Persistent, throbbing pain
- Sensitivity to hot and cold
- Pain when chewing or biting
- Swelling around the tooth

- Fever

- Bad taste in the mouth

- Swollen glands

Actions that may help:

- Press a cold compress or ice pack wrapped in a cloth against the affected area.

- Avoid lying down. Elevate your head to help reduce blood flow to the painful area and alleviate pressure on the tooth.

- Avoid food or drinks that can trigger the pain, including very hot or cold food and drinks, and hard food such as nuts.

- Maintain good oral hygiene to keep the affected tooth clean and free of debris.

HOMEOPATHIC REMEDIES

Belladonna

- **Throbbing** pain; painful **swelling of gums**; gum boil or abscess; fast, **sudden**, **intense pain**, especially **lower teeth on right side**; very sensitive to touch, **all senses acute**; dry mouth with aversion to water; swelling in affected part; **hot, red face**

- Worse at night; with **pressure**; eating; **touch**; jarring motion

- Better with **biting on something**

Chamomilla

- **Intolerable pain**; highly emotional; **oversensitive**; irritable; temperamental; **angry**; swelling of the cheek, **one side red, the other pale**; swollen, burning gums; thirsty for **cold drinks**

- Worse during **pregnancy**; during **menstruation**; for **touch**; being cold; with coffee; warm drinks; in a stuffy room; between **9 p.m. and midnight**

- Better for **cold applications**

Coffea Cruda

- **Hypersensitive jaw**; **severe, intolerable pain**; wants to rub affected part but too sensitive; **overreactive**; weepy; anxiety; **restlessness**; insomnia

- Useful for **teething** in sensitive children; toothache during **menstruation**

- Worse for **touch**; **warm drinks**; **coffee**; at night

- Better for **holding ice or cold water in mouth**; cold drinks; **lying down**; sleep

Hypericum

- **Sharp, shooting pain** along the nerve; feels like **nerve is exposed**; sensitive and painful teeth

- Useful for **injuries to nerves**

- Worse from **touch**; jarring motion

- Better for bending head backwards; **lying on affected side**

*Hypericum is a good remedy to take after
dental work, alongside Arnica.*

Mag Phos

- **Hypersensitive** to pain; screaming or **crying out**; sudden, **shooting pain**; severe **neuralgic pain** in decayed or filled teeth; **restlessness**; nervousness; **weeping**; despair; anxiety; exhaustion; fear of being touched

- Worse for **cold water**; at night; with **touch**; motion; **cold air**

- Better from **heat** and **warmth**; hard pressure; rubbing

Plantago

- **Earache**; sensitive teeth, sore to touch; **profuse salivation**; sharp, **stabbing pains that shoot to left side of face**; sharp pains in eyes

- Use for toothache in **cavities**; **decayed** or **rotten** teeth

- Worse at night; with **touch**; **heat** and **cold**

- Better when **eating**; with **sleep**

*Plantago is the number one herbal remedy
for toothache and bleeding gums.*

Pulsatilla

- Sharp, shooting pain extends to the **head**, **face** or **eye** of affected side; sensation of '**stretched nerve**'; **tearful**; wants affection and sympathy

- Worse in the evening (at **twilight**); coming into **warmth** from outside; from heat of bed coverings

- Better for **holding cold water in mouth**; cool, fresh, **open air**; **cold applications**; slow motion; being carried; **consolation**

Calc Fluor 6x

This cell salt strengthens tooth enamel, making it particularly helpful for children who are prone to getting cavities easily. When the enamel is weak, it can lead to tooth decay. Calc Fluor effective for sensitive teeth, whether the sensitivity is chronic or acute, especially after eating or touching the affected tooth. It's also beneficial for damaged, crooked or misshapen teeth. This remedy can be given to children to promote better dental health as they grow. It's often taken for periods of three to six months and is excellent for both the elderly and young children.

OTHER HOME REMEDIES

Clove oil

Clove oil is a natural antiseptic and pain reliever. In some traditions, people chew cloves to release the oil and relieve a painful tooth. To use clove oil for toothache relief, add a few drops to a carrier oil such as olive or coconut oil and apply it to the painful tooth. It's important to be cautious because pure clove oil can be irritating if not properly diluted.

Thyme mouthwash

Thyme is a natural antioxidant and antiseptic, so it can help keep the area clean. Make a mouthwash by adding a few drops of essential thyme oil to water and swishing it around the mouth and teeth. Alternatively, put a few drops onto a cotton wool pad and dab around the affected tooth.

Peppermint tea bag

A cold peppermint tea bag can help ease and numb a toothache. Steep the teabag in hot water for a minute, then remove it, let it cool and place on the affected tooth. For enhanced cooling relief, place the tea bag in the freezer before applying.

TRAVEL SICKNESS

Travel sickness, or motion sickness, is a common condition caused by signals from the inner ear to the brain that differ from those received by the eyes. It occurs during travel and is aggravated by exaggerated vehicle motion, such as the rocking of a boat or twists and turns while driving. It can be experienced on any mode of transport.

The severity of sickness varies among individuals and relief can be immediate once the journey has ended. Travel sickness is common in childhood, but most children grow out of it. It can also affect adults.

Signs of travel sickness include:

- Nausea

- Vomiting

- Dizziness

- Anxiety

- Pale and feeling cold

- Headache

Actions that may help:

- To ease sickness, choose the front seat in a car, or the centre if you're on a boat or plane, and look ahead to the horizon.

- Ensure exposure to fresh, open air, either by sitting near an open window or by a vent.

- Avoid reading or looking at a screen while travelling.

- Stay hydrated by taking regular sips of water.

- Schedule frequent stop breaks on a road trip.

HOMEOPATHIC REMEDIES

Cocculus

- **Dizziness**; fainting; **nausea**; **vomiting**; nausea at thought or smell of food; **metallic taste** in mouth; **headache**, can't lie on back of head

- Car sickness from **reading** or **looking out of the window** and **seeing a moving object**

- Worse with **lack of sleep**; eating; exertion; bending over; in **cold, open air**

- Better for sitting in a **warm room**; being **quiet**

Cocculus is the number one remedy
for motion sickness.

Petroleum

- Nausea from any kind of **rocking** or **up-and-down** motion; dizziness with **ringing in ears**, as if **intoxicated**; feels **weak** and **faint**, hypoglycaemic symptoms, **must eat**; headache, back of head

- Car, train or seasickness

- Worse for **motion**; eating; breathing **petrol fumes**

- Better for **closing eyes**; lying with **head elevated**; in open air; from **cold water on face**

Tabacum

- Sudden **loss of energy**; **pale** or green; vertigo; **cold sweats**; nausea; vomiting; **sinking feeling** in stomach

- Seasickness or car sickness

- Worse in **confined spaces**

- Better for fresh, open air, with **cold applications**; with **abdomen uncovered**

OTHER HOME REMEDIES

Ginger

Ginger has extensive digestive health benefits and can help with travel sickness, too. It can relieve the nausea and vomiting associated with motion during travelling. To settle the stomach, start taking ginger 30 minutes before the journey begins and consume it as needed. Prepare ginger tea using slices of the fresh root, take ginger capsules or eat crystallized ginger.

Lemon or lime

The strong scent or taste of lemons or limes can alleviate motion sickness. Suck on a slice of lemon or lime during a journey or add their juice to a bottle of water. Another option is to put a few drops of essential lemon oil on a cloth and inhale the scent to help settle the stomach.

Plugging an ear

This method reportedly works for some to prevent seasickness: blocking one ear with an earplug. This causes the brain to perceive a hearing issue, causing it to ignore conflicting sensory information.

WARTS AND VERRUCAS

Warts

Common warts are especially prevalent in children and are thought to be caused by a virus. Some children are more susceptible to warts than others. Common warts are contagious and can be passed through direct contact or by touching objects or surfaces that an infected person has touched. Although they do go away on their own, it can take up to two years for them to disappear completely.

Signs of warts include:

- Small, flesh-coloured bumps that vary in size
- Can have a rough or bumpy texture and look like a small cauliflower
- Can be single or in clusters
- Found on knees, hands, thumbs and fingers
- Not painful, but can itch or bleed if knocked

Actions that may help:

- Avoid touching the warts to prevent the spread of them to other parts of the body.
- Maintain good hygiene.

- To prevent the spread of the virus, avoid biting fingernails if the warts are on the fingers.

- Eat a healthy, wholefood diet, exercise regularly and sleep well to support the immune system.

Verrucas

Verrucas, also known as plantar warts, are found on the feet and can be painful when pressure is directly applied, e.g. when walking or standing. They may be flat or raised with thickened skin.

Signs of a verruca include:

- Found on the weight-bearing areas of the foot: the heels, soles or balls of the feet

- Can be surrounded by thickened skin (callus)

- Size can vary from pinhead-sized bumps to large growths

- Normally flesh-coloured with tiny black dots within the verruca

Actions that may help:

- Maintain good foot hygiene, keeping feet clean and dry to avoid moist conditions.

- Change socks regularly, especially if feet tend to sweat excessively.

- Wear footwear in communal areas such as swimming pools, gyms and changing rooms.

- Avoid sharing towels, shoes and socks.

HOMEOPATHIC REMEDIES

Ant Crud

- Hard, **smooth verrucas**, often in groups and on **soles of feet**; ragged growths; **horny warts**, rough, scaly skin growths with hard, horn-like surface, tender and **painful to walk on**; **digestive issues** from overeating; **white-coated tongue**

Nitric-ac

- Large, jagged warts; itchy, moist, cauliflower-like warts; warts **bleed on touch** or after washing; warts on **back of hands**

Silica

- **Unhealthy-looking skin**; abscesses or wart-like growths; **delayed healing** of skin eruptions, don't disappear; fragile, **dry hair**; **flaking nails**; offensive-smelling sweat, particularly from feet

Thuja

- Warts, polyps and molluscum after **vaccinations**; wart-like eruptions that **itch**; eruptions only on **covered areas** of body; chronic **thick, green mucus** in nose or coughing up

OTHER HOME REMEDIES

Apple cider vinegar

As a well-known remedy for killing microbes such as viruses and fungi, apple cider vinegar breaks down the hard layers of skin produced by a wart. Soak a pad or gauze in apple cider vinegar and secure it using a bandage or plaster; leave it on overnight. Repeat every night for 10 to 14 days. Dilute the apple cider vinegar if it irritates the surrounding skin.

Garlic

Garlic, with its antiviral properties, can be effective in treating warts. Crush a garlic clove and mix with a few drops of water to make a paste. Apply the paste to the wart, secure it using a plaster and leave it overnight. Wash off and repeat nightly until the wart has gone.

Banana peel

A common home remedy is using a banana peel to break down the hard layers of a wart. Cut a piece of banana peel and fix the inside of the skin against the wart with a bandage or plaster. Leave this on overnight and repeat until the wart has gone. Alternatively, rub the area with the peel morning and night.

HOMEOPATHIC
REMEDY KIT

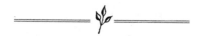

Homeopathy is fun to use and easy to learn. Even a beginner can make a big difference in resolving common complaints, such as minor cuts and bruises, with a few remedies.

Learning how homeopathic remedies work will increase your confidence and help you when dealing with other health issues. Most people experience similar symptoms after minor injuries, making it simple to discover which remedy to use for each condition.

As you become more confident, start using homeopathic remedies for complaints such as coughs, colds and headaches. It's important to tailor the remedy to the individual's symptoms rather than the cause of the complaint. Remember the CLAMS method (*see page xxii*). Colds, for instance, vary from one season to the next and from person to person. As a result, the remedies that are needed will also differ, and you need to learn to choose between them.

Homeopathic remedies are relatively inexpensive, long-lasting and safe for all ages. They're also easy to obtain. Many common ones are available online, in natural health stores, pharmacies and sometimes even supermarkets. Use the list below to help you build your own homeopathic first aid kit.

Top 10 homeopathic remedies for the home

1. Aconite

- Good remedy for **beginning** of acute illness or infection; for **shock**, such as from **fright** or bad news; for acute conditions with **sudden onset**, such as sore throats, headaches or croup – typically **childhood** complaints

- **Intense thirst** for cold drinks; **great fear** or **anxiety**; **restlessness**; intolerable pain; feeling chilled after exposure to **dry**, **cold winds** or draughts

- Worse around **midnight**; after fright or shock; in a confined, warm room

- Better in fresh, **open air**; from sitting still

2. Apis Mel

- Good remedy for **insect bites** or **stings**, and **allergic reactions**, e.g. hives; **cystitis** with frequent urination, **burning** and **stinging** pain; shingles and **urticaria** with large, raised, white, **itchy** bumps

- **Red**, **hot**, inflamed and **swollen** affected area; burning and stinging pain; **thirstless**

- Worse with **heat**; **touch**; lying down; at night; after sleep; with pressure; in a closed room

- Better for **cool**, **fresh air**; having **cold drinks**; changing position

3. Arnica

- Good remedy for **trauma, injury** and **bruising** to muscles and soft tissues; for individuals who avoid attention, insist they're okay, but may be in shock; for conditions that leave individuals feeling **sore, as if beaten**, or who are **restless** and can't get comfortable; for jet lag

- Can be taken **before or after surgery, dental work** or **childbirth** to prevent trauma and bruising

- Worse with **touch**; pressure; **jarring motion**; after sleep

- Better for **lying down**; changing position; **cold baths**; in **open air**; with **loose-fitting clothes**

4. Arsenicum Album

- Good remedy for **digestion issues**, e.g. food poisoning with diarrhoea and vomiting

- **Weakness; very chilly; anxious about health** and disease; **restlessness**; exhaustion; insomnia; **burning** pain and discharges; thirsty for cold water but **sips only**

- Worse with **cold**; around **midnight** (between 11 p.m. and 2 a.m.)

- Better for **heat**; company; sitting up; elevating head; in open air

5. Belladonna

- Good remedy for acute conditions that appear **suddenly**, then disappear as quickly; for the **start of an infection**; for **fevers**, sunstroke, **headaches**; for any infections that produce boils or abscesses

- Inflammation and **redness**; fast, **sudden**, **intense**, shooting or **throbbing** pain; sensation of blood rushing to one area, a feeling of **congestion**; affected part **radiates heat**; red, **flushed face**; **glassy eyes**; very sensitive to pain; wants to be wrapped up; **craves lemons** and lemonade

- Worse for movement; with **touch**; being heated; jarring motion; exposure to **draughts**; light; around **3 p.m.**

- Better for standing; sitting upright; **bending backwards**; being in a **warm room**

6. Gelsemium

- Good remedy for influenza; ailments from **bad news**; states of **shock** like 'rabbit in the headlights'; apprehension, anticipation and **dread of new situations**, exams or presentations

- Gradual onset of symptoms; feels paralysed; physical and emotional **weakness**; **trembling** from fright or anticipation; **drowsiness**; **apathy**; headache, like a **tight band** around head; **droopy eyelids**; **thirstless**

- Worse from **mental exertion**; sun exposure; lying down

- Better for pressure; head elevated in bed; **urination**

7. Hepar Sulph

- Good remedy for abscesses, boils, croup, colds, ear infections and tonsillitis; for aliments from **getting chilled** or sitting in a dry, cold draught

- Inflammation; **yellow**, **thick**, **foul-smelling pus** like **old cheese**; **splinter-like**, stabbing pain; very chilly; **irritable**; **oversensitive**

- Worse from cold; **slightest draught**; touch; in open air; on waking
- Better in damp weather; with heat; from **wrapping up**

8. Hypericum

- Good remedy for insect **stings** and animal **bites** with a **puncture** wound; **lacerated** wounds where there is tearing of the flesh; injuries to **nerve-rich areas**, e.g. fingers, spine; whiplash and **neck injuries**; injuries to **coccyx**; **crushed fingers**; after root canal **dental work** and **surgery**

- More tender than appearance would suggest; sharp, **shooting pains**; **radiating pain**

- Worse from **cold**; **damp**; with touch; **pressure**

- Better for **rubbing** affected areas; for warmth

9. Nux Vomica

- Good remedy for **hangover** headaches, nausea and vomiting; **digestive issues**, e.g. stomach upsets and **indigestion**; complaints from **overindulging** in **rich food**, drinking alcohol and coffee, and taking recreational **drugs**

- **Irritability; impatience; anger**; mental strain; **constipation** with haemorrhoids; insomnia from **work worries**

- Worse in the **morning**; with **cold**; **alcohol**; **noise**; tight-fitting clothes

- Better with **heat**; lying down; hot drinks; naps

10. Rhus Tox

- Good remedy for **sprains** and **strains** of muscles or tendons; injuries from **overexertion**, e.g. exercise, gardening or straining voice; acute pain of rheumatism, arthritis or sciatica; influenza with stiffness and soreness; skin rashes like chicken pox and shingles, with **red**, **hot**, **itchy blisters**

- **Stiffness**; **pain**; **restlessness**

- Worse with first movement; cold; **damp**, wet weather; getting wet; at night

- Better with continued movement; **heat**; hot baths; changing position

Ointments, creams and tinctures to have at home

Arnica cream

Arnica cream is a great remedy for various minor injuries and ailments. One of its main benefits is its ability to reduce swelling and bruising. When applied to an affected area, it helps to soothe muscle pain and stiffness, making it particularly useful for sprains, strains and other soft tissue injuries.

It's a convenient remedy for anyone with an active lifestyle or those engaging in physical activities that can result in minor injuries. For example, after a long run or a strenuous workout, muscles can feel sore and achy. Applying Arnica cream can provide much-needed relief by reducing inflammation and promoting faster healing.

Arnica cream is very easy to use; simply apply a small amount to the affected area and gently massage it. With regular application, it helps to prevent the development of bruising and can significantly reduce the discomfort associated with minor injuries. It's important not to apply the cream to broken skin, as it can irritate.

Calendula cream

Calendula cream is an excellent remedy to keep in your first aid kit. Its healing and anti-inflammatory properties make it particularly useful for various skin issues. Here are some key indications for using Calendula cream:

- Minor cuts and scrapes: Ensure the wound is clean and free of dirt or foreign bodies. Then apply a thin layer of cream to help speed up the healing process and prevent infection.

- Its anti-inflammatory properties help reduce redness and promote healing, soothing minor burns and sunburn.

- It provides relief and promotes healing for skin irritations and rashes, including nappy rash in babies. It's gentle enough for sensitive skin, making it suitable for children and adults.

- Calendula can be beneficial for healing post-surgical wounds.

- Eczema and dermatitis: Regular application can provide ongoing relief in chronic conditions, helping to soothe the skin and reduce inflammation.

- Applying Calendula cream to insect bites and stings can provide quick relief, helping reduce itching and swelling.

Calendula tincture

Calendula tincture is excellent for treating minor wounds, cuts and abrasions. It can be used to gently bathe the affected area by diluting it in boiled and cooled or sterile water. Cleaning the site and reducing the chance of infection will support the body's natural healing. Additionally, it's beneficial after dental work or childbirth, where it can be used as a soothing rinse to aid in recovery and comfort. The choice between Calendula tincture and Calendula cream depends on the nature of the wound or condition.

Hyper Cal cream

This cream can be applied directly to the skin, especially for wounds that are in the process of healing or for less severe skin issues like minor cuts, abrasions or stinging pains. It combines the healing properties of Calendula with the pain-relieving properties of Hypericum, making it a great option for promoting rapid healing and providing antiseptic protection. It's also easier to apply and less messy than the tincture solution (*see below*).

Hyper Cal tincture

This form is particularly useful for cleaning and bathing wounds. For a cut, abrasion or any open wound, dilute the tincture in cooled boiled water. This solution acts as an antiseptic, helping clean the wound and promote healing while providing pain relief. It's especially beneficial for wounds that are sensitive to touch or have a lot of nerve involvement, as the Hypericum component is excellent for nerve pain.

A–Z OF HOMEOPATHIC REMEDIES

This book discusses two types of remedies: tablets or capsules for internal use, and ointments, creams and herbal tinctures for external use.

RESOURCES

Scan the QR code below to visit my online digital diagnostic tool 'Ask Marcus', where you can ask me any question about home prescribing:

Scan the QR code below to receive your FREE online course on Home Prescribing:

For more online and classroom courses from beginner to practitioner level, visit: www.chehomeopathy.com

Where to purchase homeopathic remedies

UK

- Ainsworths Homoeopathic Pharmacy: www.ainsworths.com

- Helios Homeopathic Pharmacies: www.helios.co.uk

- Freemans Homeopathic Pharmacy: www.freemans.scot

- The Centre for Homeopathic Education (CHE): www.chehomeopathy.com/remedies

- Weleda: www.weleda.co.uk

USA

- Hahnemann Labs: www.hahnemannlabs.com

- Washington Homeopathic Products: www.homeopathyworks. com

Canada

- Thompson's Homeopathic Supplies Ltd.: www.thompsonshomeopathic.com

Australia

- Eugénie Krüger Homeopathy: www.eugeniekruger.com

- Martin & Pleasance: www.martinandpleasance.com

- The Family Apothecary: www.thefamilyapothecary.com.au

Professional homeopathic organizations

UK

- Homeopathy International: www.hint.org.uk

- The Society of Homeopaths: www.homeopathy-soh.org

- The Alliance of Registered Homeopaths: www.a-r-h.org

- British Association of Homeopathic Veterinary Surgeons: www.bahvs.net

- British Homeopathic Dental Association: www.bhda.co.uk

USA

- National Center for Homeopathy: www.homeopathycenter.org

- North American Society of Homeopaths: www.homeopathy.org

Canada

- Canadian Society of Homeopaths: www.csoh.ca

Australia

- Australian Homeopathic Association (AHA): www.homeopathyoz.org

- The Australian Register of Homoeopaths (AROH): www.aroh.com.au

ACKNOWLEDGEMENTS

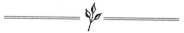

Throughout my homoeopathic journey, which spans over three decades, I have been inspired by numerous remarkable individuals.

I want to express my heartfelt appreciation to the late, great Robert Davidson, who first opened my young mind to a revolutionary perspective on health and wellbeing. He ignited within me a passion to approach homeopathy with fearlessness and enthusiasm.

I have profound gratitude and thanks to the late, great Dr Robin Murphy, who graciously took me under his wing when I was a young student of homeopathy. He became a lifelong mentor, teacher and good friend. He taught me the importance of keeping it simple and showed me that homeopathy *is* the medicine of the people.

To all the students and graduates from the Centre for Homeopathic Education (CHE) around the world: Your zeal for learning and love for homeopathy have transformed teaching into one of the most fulfilling experiences imaginable for me.

To the dedicated staff and lecturers at CHE: Your expertise, passion and tireless efforts have shaped countless homeopaths and advanced our field. Your commitment to excellence and innovative teaching has created an environment where homeopathy thrives, and I'm honoured to work alongside such devoted professionals.

To my patients and clients: You have taught me invaluable lessons about homeopathy and the body's innate ability to heal.

I extend my sincere gratitude to Hay House for providing me with the opportunity to share this wonderful healing modality with others who are looking for a more natural way to treat themselves and their families.

A special thanks to my editor, Nicola, whose patience and dedication to this project have been invaluable. Your meticulous work and insights have significantly enhanced this book.

To my children, Jimmy and Maggie: Thank you for bringing fun, laughter and joy into my life and for bestowing upon me the precious gift of fatherhood.

And to my beloved wife, Emma: Words cannot express the depth of my gratitude for your unwavering love, endless patience, steadfast support and profound understanding throughout our 30-year journey together. Your presence by my side has not only made this path infinitely easier to traverse, but has also imbued it with a sense of fulfilment and purpose that I could never have achieved alone.

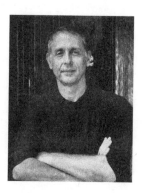

ABOUT THE AUTHOR

Marcus Fernandez has been involved in homeopathy for more than 30 years and has practised and taught all over the world. In 1998, along with two colleagues, he founded the Centre for Homeopathic Education (CHE), the largest school of homeopathy in the UK.

As the Principal and founder of CHE, his aim is to enhance the health and wellbeing of humankind through the education and application of homeopathy.

He passionately believes the more that people use homeopathy in the home, the more they will become empowered to take charge of their health and the health of their families.

In 2021, Marcus was made a Fellow of the Society of Homeopaths for his outstanding contribution to homeopathy.

www.marcus-fernandez.com

NOTES

We hope you enjoyed this Hay House book. If you'd like to receive our online catalog featuring additional information on Hay House books and products, or if you'd like to find out more about the Hay Foundation, please contact:

Hay House LLC, P.O. Box 5100, Carlsbad, CA 92018-5100
(760) 431-7695 or (800) 654-5126
www.hayhouse.com® • www.hayfoundation.org

―――

Published in Australia by:
Hay House Australia Publishing Pty Ltd
18/36 Ralph St., Alexandria NSW 2015
Phone: +61 (02) 9669 4299
www.hayhouse.com.au

Published in the United Kingdom by:
Hay House UK Ltd
1st Floor, Crawford Corner,
91–93 Baker Street, London W1U 6QQ
Phone: +44 (0)20 3927 7290
www.hayhouse.co.uk

Published in India by:
Hay House Publishers (India) Pvt Ltd
Muskaan Complex, Plot No. 3,
B-2, Vasant Kunj, New Delhi 110 070
Phone: +91 11 41761620
www.hayhouse.co.in

―――

Let Your Soul Grow

Experience life-changing transformation—one video
at a time—with guidance from the world's leading experts.

www.healyourlifeplus.com